BEYO

THE

SURGERY

Life After Fibroids.

Beating the Odds through Nutrition

NINA LEMTIR

DEDICATION

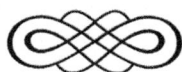

To my three beautiful children, **Vanea, Silverlyn-Rose**, and **Harvey** you are my light, my strength, and the reason I continue to strive for greatness. Your love inspires me every day.

To my mum, **Roseline Lawir**, whose unwavering support, and wisdom have guided me through life's toughest challenges thank you for your unconditional love and belief in me.

To my incredible sisters, **Beri** and **Bernadette** your encouragement, laughter, and sisterhood have been a source of endless comfort and joy.

And to my amazing clients, whose bravery and commitment to their healing journeys continue to inspire me. Thank you for trusting me to walk alongside you as you reclaim your health and power.

This book is for all of you. Thank you for being my foundation, my motivation, and my greatest blessings.

TABLE OF CONTENTS

ACKNOWLEDGMENTS

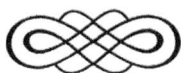

This book, *Beyond The Surgery*, would not have been possible without the love, guidance, and support of so many incredible individuals.

First and foremost, I thank my family for their unwavering encouragement and patience as I navigated this journey. To my children, you are my inspiration, my joy, and my constant reminder of why perseverance matters.

To the countless women who shared their stories and struggles with me—your courage and resilience have shaped every word of this book. Thank you for trusting me with your truth and fueling my passion to create hope and healing.

To my mentors and colleagues in holistic health and wellness, your wisdom and shared experiences have been invaluable in crafting the practical strategies within these pages.

To my editor and publishing team, thank you for your tireless efforts, keen insights, and belief in the power of this message. Your dedication ensured that this book became everything I dreamed it could be.

And finally, to God, for the strength and clarity to transform pain into purpose, and for reminding me that every challenge is a stepping stone to something greater.

This book is for every woman who has felt silenced, overlooked, or trapped in repetitive surgery on her health journey. Together, we are rewriting the narrative and reclaiming our power.

With gratitude,

Nina Lemtir

FOREWORD

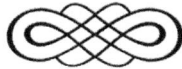

As an Obstetrician and Gynaecologist with a particular passion for equitable care for women and girls it is with great pleasure that I write this foreword. When I was introduced to Nina by Bernie Davies, the visionary force behind Mastering Diversity, I felt an instant kinship; a shared vision for facilitating women to become empowered partners in their healthcare experiences. As a Black woman myself I understand that current healthcare systems are not designed with us in mind and the intersectionality of race and gender have led to our exclusion from the voices shaping Gynaecological services. There are few things more impactful than the patient's story in motivating change and I applaud Nina's courage in stepping forward to tell hers with such vulnerability and honesty. Nina's story is a powerful example of how a simple change to listening and understanding the concerns and needs of the women in our care can transform their lives.

It is estimated that 8 in 10 Black women will experience fibroids by the age of 50, and yet there is little readily available information to empower these women to feel able advocate for their care needs. *Beyond The Surgery* is a very welcome addition to this space. The societal normalisation of pain and clinicians' diminishment of heavy menstrual bleeding is an all-too-common narrative, leaving women distrustful of healthcare providers and isolated in managing their often-debilitating symptoms.

This story of Nina's lived experience of navigating through the labyrinth of Women's healthcare is an essential read for clinicians working in women's health, women undertaking their own menstrual health journeys and their loved ones supporting them. She highlights the importance of collaborative decision making and the reality of the disparities in care for women from marginalised groups, where bias and misconceptions result in poorer outcomes. The surgical options routinely offered for management of fibroids are often invasive and potentially fertility-limiting, leaving women forced to make the unbearable decision between quality of life and motherhood. Nina's well researched message around the newly recognised importance of holistic and individualised care, with explanation of the impact of chronic stress and suboptimal nutrition on gynaecological health, reflects the need for us all to make a change and look *Beyond The Surgery*.

"The greatest medicine of all is teaching people how not to need it."- Hippocrates.

Dr Tipswalo Day: Award Winning Obstetrician and Gynaecologist at Glangwili General Hospital, Wales, Advocate, humanitarian.

CHAPTER 1

UNDERSTANDING FIBROIDS AND MYOMECTOMY

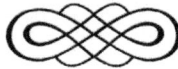

The Basics of Uterine Fibroids

Hello, my dear reader. First, let me thank you for picking up this book. Before we dive into a whole world of fibroids, surgeries, and holistic healing, let me tell you a bit about myself and my journey, because this is not just a book about a condition; it is about real life, real pain, and real hope.

My name is Nina, and my story begins in the beautiful, vibrant country of Cameroon, located in West Africa—a land rich in culture and history, colonised by both the

French and the English. I come from the English-speaking region called Kumbo, a place where dreams are big, and challenges are met with resilience.

At the tender age of one, my journey took a new turn. My mum and dad made the brave decision to migrate to the UK in search of a better life, bringing me along with them (which was a last minute decision). We became part of a small, close-knit community of Cameroonian migrants living in the iconic location of Tower Bridge in London,. Navigating the complexities of a new country while holding tightly to our roots and traditions was as exciting as it was challenging back then.

As a little girl, I dreamed of many things: running my own successful salon, building a loving family, and living a vibrant, healthy life. For a while, those dreams felt so close, so attainable—until they were not. My journey took unexpected turns, filled with challenges I never imagined, but it also shaped the woman I am today.

Growing up, I was no stranger to the sharp sting of words and the isolating feeling of being "different." My childhood took a dark turn when my mum became a single mother. She carried immense pressures on her shoulders, doing everything she could to provide for us while battling the trials of life alone. Those pressures did not just weigh on her; they filtered through to me in ways I could not understand at the time.

Food became my solace, and constant companion. It was there for me when the world felt overwhelming, offering comfort when I needed it most. But over time, that respite came with a cost, as the weight slowly began to pile on.

As a teenager, I was often bullied for being overweight. The whispered insults, the pointed laughter in hallways, and the cruel remarks etched themselves into my mind. Each taunt felt like another stone added to the weight I was already carrying.

Those experiences could have easily defined me, shaping my identity around the harsh words and ridicule. But I refused to let them. They became the fuel that drove me to dig deeper, to find strength within myself, and to rise above the pain.

Despite the emotional toll of bullying, I found my place in academics. I learned early on that my worth was not tied to the superficial judgments of others but to the strength of my resolve. I poured my energy into my studies, using my achievements as a shield against the negativity. My goals carved a path for me that burned brighter than the weight of their taunts.

When the day came, standing on the stage to receive my first-class degree was not just a triumph of intellect but a testament to resilience. I was validated. It was proof that the girl they tried to diminish could rise above it all, propelled by the very challenges that sought to defeat her.

This milestone was the first step toward reclaiming my power. Those years taught me that adversity could either be a stumbling block or a stepping stone. I chose to use it as a platform to push myself towards my dreams. Little did I know that this inner strength, forged during my youth, would become my most valuable ally in the battles yet to come.

The first signs that something was wrong crept quietly in. At first, they were just "annoying" inconveniences, cramps that were a little worse than usual, periods that seemed to last forever. I would brush them off, thinking I was simply overworked. My career was thriving; I was building something of which I was proud. But as the symptoms grew worse, they began to overshadow everything I loved. I started feeling tired, bone-deep exhaustion that sleep could not fix. My clothes no longer fit as my abdomen inexplicably swelled. There were days I could not stand up straight as the pain gripped me so fiercely.

Yet, like many women, I soldiered on, afraid to admit just how bad it was. Like most of us, I was taught to push through pain, to never let weakness show. Watching my mum look after us as a single mum, I cannot recall her going to the doctors. She just seemed to always get on with life without complaints. And so, I ignored my body's cries for help, until I could not anymore.

The diagnosis was devastating: fibroids. And not just any fibroids, but ones that had grown large enough to distort my womb (the size of a 7 month pregnancy), and affecting my ability to have children. My heart shattered into a million pieces. How could this be happening to me? I had always envisioned myself as a mother. And now, not only was that dream slipping away, but the life I had built felt as though it was crumbling beneath me.

The treatment options I was presented with were brutal: invasive surgery, hormonal treatments with severe side effects, or, as some doctors hinted, simply accepting a hysterectomy as part of the process of trying to address the problem. "It's the only way to solve this," they said.

I remember sitting in sterile hospital rooms, feeling like a number, not a person. There was no empathy, no understanding—just cold, clinical facts.

Outside of the doctor's office, the reactions were mixed. Some friends and family offered support, but others dismissed my struggles. "At least it's not cancer," they said, as if that made the daily suffering any less.

Others told me to "just get on with it" or suggested that I was exaggerating. The lack of understanding was isolating, and I began to feel like I was screaming into a void.

But somewhere in the depths of despair, a spark ignited. I was not ready to give up on myself or my dreams. I refused to accept that surgery or suffering were my only options. I pleaded with the consultant to consider not removing all of the fibroids, as what I understood was that severe blood loss during the operation would increase the chances of them having to perform a hysterectomy. That was not an option for me. So if we cut the operating time, surely my chances to keep my uterus would increase. They subsequently agreed to my request and I got through the procedure by the grace of God. It was very touch and go as I had bled heavily.

Sitting in the sterile, impersonal office of the consultant, I felt a knot tighten in my stomach as the words I had dreaded were finally spoken. "There's a high chance the fibroids will grow back," the doctor said, matter-of-factly. "If you want to conceive, you need to try sooner rather than later."

The air suddenly sucked from the room. My mind raced, filled with questions I did not know how to voice. How soon? How much time did I really have? And what if I did not conceive? Was this a gamble I was destined to lose? The very idea of trying to create life under such immense pressure felt extremely overwhelming.

But the consultant's words were deafeningly clear…devoid of any sugarcoating: my clock was ticking faster than I could have imagined. I was caught between two daunting realities—the potential return of the fibroids and continued growth of the existing ones, and the uncertainty of whether my body could sustain a pregnancy at all. It felt like an ultimatum with no clear alternative.

I left that appointment, my mind fraught with a mix of determination and fear. I understood the medical reasoning, but the emotional toll was immense. I realised then that I was not just fighting fibroids—I was also battling the onset of time, expectation, and the haunting possibilities…the "what ifs."

This moment marked a turning point in my journey, one that fueled my resolve to approach my health with a new sense of urgency and empowerment. I remember sitting in the sterile, impersonal office of yet another consultant, hearing the words that should have shattered me: "You may have to accept that motherhood might not be in your future."

For a few moments, time seemed to stop. The room, the voices—it all became a blur. But then, as if a light flickered on inside me, I recalled something I had seen just days before: a woman on social media sharing her story of overcoming seemingly unprecedented odds, defying the limits doctors had placed on her. Her courage resonated deeply with me, sparking a small but undeniable flame within me.

I realised then that I had a choice. I could surrender to the despair of those words, or I could rewrite my narrative. No consultant's prognosis would dictate the hope I held for my future. That singular memory—her resilience and determination—became the catalyst for mine.

From that day forward, I resolved to take control of my story. I would educate myself, make the necessary lifestyle changes, and approach my health with a fierceness that mirrored the hope I carried. I decided that no matter what the odds, I would take control of my story— because no consultant's outlook could dictate the hope I held for my future.

I immediately launched my search for alternative paths to healing. I devoured books, sought out experts, changed careers and immersed myself in learning about the root causes of cell dysfunctions and fibroids and how the body could heal itself with the right tools. I boldly made the difficult decision to close my salon as I needed to focus entirely on my healing.

This journey was not easy. I stumbled, doubted, and sometimes wanted to give up. But I pressed on, experimenting with nutrition, lifestyle changes, and emotional healing. Slowly but surely, I began to see results. My body started responding; the swelling reduced, the pain lessened, and my energy returned. I went from barely surviving to truly thriving.

Now, as I sit writing here to you, I want you to know this: you are not alone. I have been where you are scared, frustrated, and unsure of what lies ahead. But there is hope. Through this book, I want to share everything I have learned about healing fibroids and reclaiming your life. It is not just about shrinking fibroids; it is about rediscovering your power and living the life you deserve.

So, let us take this journey together. Think of this book as a conversation between friends—a place where you can find understanding, guidance, and inspiration. In the next chapters, we will go into more detail about what fibroids are, why they develop, and how you can take control of your healing. But for now, take a deep breath and know this: you are stronger than you think, and your story is far from over.

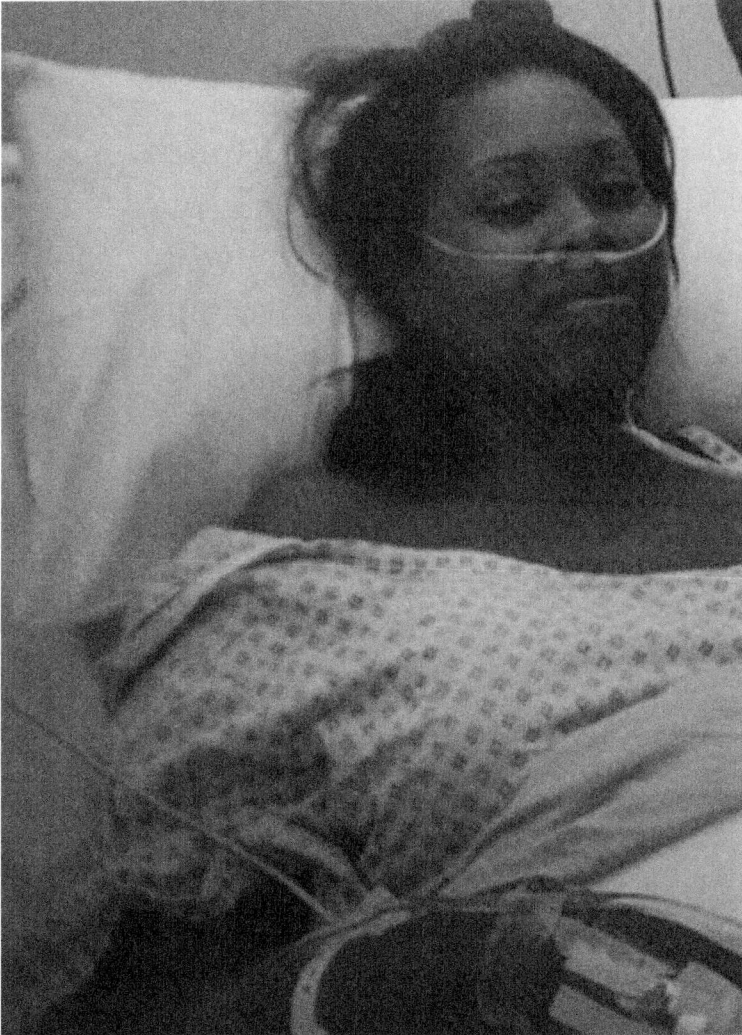

Let us begin.

Uterine fibroids are non-cancerous growths that develop in or on the uterus, affecting a significant number of women during their reproductive years. For professional and entrepreneurial women, understanding the basics of fibroids is crucial, as they impact not only physical health but also emotional well-being and productivity. These growths vary in size and number, often causing symptoms such as heavy menstrual bleeding, infertility, pelvic pain, and pressure, although sometimes they can be asymptomatic. Knowing what fibroids are and how they develop is the first step toward taking control of your health, and fertility. Making informed decisions, through research and acting on what affects your body is vital.

The exact cause of uterine fibroids remains unclear, but research suggests that hormonal factors, particularly estrogen and progesterone, play a significant role in their growth. These hormones stimulate the uterine lining and contribute to the development of fibroids during a woman's reproductive years. Genetic factors and lifestyle choices, including nutrition and stress management, also significantly influence fibroid development and growth. As you embrace a holistic approach to your womb and overall health, it is key to recognise that lifestyle modifications create a supportive environment for your body, mind, and soul, reducing the likelihood of fibroid recurrence after invasive or less invasive surgery.

After undergoing a myomectomy, it is essential to adopt a proactive approach to nutrition and lifestyle to prevent the regrowth of fibroids and other potential complications from the procedure. **As adhesions are extremely prevalent in postoperative pelvic adhesions and occur in 25% to 92% of patients undergoing abdominal surgery (Okabayashi et al., 2014). With a myomectomy being the most adhesiogenic procedure (Keckstein et al., 1994).** A well-balanced diet rich in low sugary fruits, vegetables, whole grains, and organic lean proteins help to regulate hormone levels and minimise inflammation consistently. Incorporating foods that are high in fibre and antioxidants support overall reproductive health and promote healing from a cellular level. Additionally, maintaining a healthy weight also further reduces the risk of fibroid recurrence, as obesity has been linked to increased estrogen levels that encourage fibroid growth.

Stress management is another critical aspect of preventing fibroid regrowth that is often overlooked. Professional women often juggle multiple responsibilities, which appears to lead to chronic stress that adversely affects hormonal balance, particularly overtime. Implementing stress-reducing practices such as yoga, spa visits, meditation, or mindfulness empowers you to take control of your mental and emotional health. These practices not only help alleviate stress but also foster a positive mindset that is essential for recovery and overall well-being. Remember this, awareness is everything in your fight against fibroids. Embracing a balanced lifestyle will empower you to thrive beyond your myomectomy, enhancing both your personal and professional life. Your success cycles will propel you to higher achievements on your healing journey. Believe that you will overcome and you will.

In your journey toward fibroid-free living, it is important to seek support and connect with other women who share similar experiences. Engage with healthcare professionals who understand your unique needs and do not accept them shrugging off your complaints. Make sure your concerns are not only documented but actioned and keep notes via a journal (digital and physical). As a professional woman, consider joining support groups focused on fibroid recovery. By actively participating in your health journey and making informed daily dietary positive choices, you will pave the way for a future free of fibroids with confidence and clarity. Develop your DMO (daily method of operation) and stick to it. Remember, your health is your greatest asset, and by prioritising it, you are investing in your ability to succeed in all areas of life. Even if you are going through a life changing event such as a divorce like myself.

The end of my marriage was more than a personal heartbreak; it was a mirror reflecting the imbalance in every corner of my life, including my health. I realised I had been so consumed by the needs of others, the stress of my responsibilities, and the weight of expectations that I had neglected the one thing I could not afford to lose: *myself.*

In the midst of the turmoil, I knew I had two choices— let this life-changing event break me or use it as the fuel to rebuild. The decision to rebuild started with a deep commitment to my health. I had to develop my DMO (daily method of operation) and stick to it relentlessly. It was a system not just for healing my body but for regaining control of my life.

Every morning, I reminded myself that my health was my greatest asset—my foundation for everything else I wanted to achieve. By prioritising it, I was investing in my ability to succeed in every area of life, even while enduring the pain and uncertainty of divorce.

Looking back, I see now that the divorce was more than just an ending; it was the catalyst for a new beginning. It taught me that even in the face of life's greatest challenges, we have the power to choose how we move forward. And for me, that choice started with taking back my health and redefining my story.

Life has not been easy, but I have stayed committed to my holistic processes. They have been my anchor, helping me navigate through the storm with more grace and clarity than I ever thought possible. I realised that how you process emotional circumstances directly impacts your health either short term or long term.

Divorce, especially when it is bitter, can leave you feeling like you have lost control. Add to that the immense responsibility of raising three children on your own, and it is easy to feel overwhelmed and stretched thin. For a while, I felt that weight too. There were days when I wanted to give up, when the stress seemed too much to bear.

But my holistic practices reminded me to take things one moment at a time. Through meditation, bio-hacking routine, and mindfulness, I learned to quiet the noise in my mind and stay present for my children and myself. The simple act of deep breathing became my go-to when emotions flared or life felt chaotic.

Nutrition also played a huge role in keeping me grounded and my body engaged. I stuck to a balanced, nourishing diet that supported my physical and emotional health, even on the toughest days. My herbal teas, nutrient-rich meals, and healing rituals helped me stay energised and calm, no matter what challenges arose.

Most importantly, these holistic tools allowed me to focus on what truly matters. They helped me let go of bitterness and redirect my energy toward building a peaceful, loving environment for my kids and myself. I realised that while I could not change the past or control other people's actions, I could control how I showed up for myself and my family. My determining factors, which is all that mattered.

Being a single mother is no easy task, but with my holistic processes, I have found a sense of balance and empowerment. They have taught me that taking care of myself is not selfish, it is essential. By staying calm and centered, I am better able to support and keep my body more in balance. Every day is a new opportunity to heal, grow, and prioritise what is important: our well-being, our dreams, and the love we share as a family. And for that, I am eternally grateful for the tools and practices that have kept me on this path.

I remember I worked tirelessly to build my hair salon from the ground up. It was my passion, my dream, and soon it became my livelihood. My salon grew from a tiny, barely noticed business into a bustling, successful enterprise of which I was incredibly proud. But the success came at a steep price. As the demands of running a busy salon increased, I found myself sacrificing more and more of my time, my energy, and eventually, my health.

Every day, I gave everything I had to my clients, focusing entirely on making them feel their best while leaving nothing for myself. I had no time for stress relief, no room for self-care. I would brush off headaches, shrug away exhaustion, and ignore nagging pain because, to me, there simply was not enough time to pause. Visiting the doctor felt impossible I was "too busy" to be sick, to take time off, or even to acknowledge that my body was crying out for help.

What I did not know was that my body had been quietly battling fibroids. I had no idea that the persistent, sometimes debilitating symptoms I was experiencing were due to these tumours. I downplayed everything, pushed through the pain, and forced myself to keep going. Even as I began experiencing deep personal losses, the miscarriages I suffered, I could not allow myself to slow down or explore what was happening.

It was after losing two pregnancies that I finally faced the truth. The losses were devastating, and as I searched for answers, I was finally diagnosed with fibroids. Hearing that word confirmed what my body had been trying to tell me all along. Yet even then, I hesitated. I had a deep seated fear of medical establishments, a fear I had carried for years. Instead of addressing the diagnosis head on, I avoided it. The fear of medical procedures, and perhaps, even of the truth itself, kept me from acting.

Looking back, I can see how I sacrificed myself for the success of my business. I poured my heart and soul into creating a thriving salon, yet in doing so, I overlooked the one person who needed my care and attention the most myself. My story is a testament to the reality that sometimes success comes with unseen costs and the journey toward healing often begins with a willingness to face our fears.

Overcoming the Odds After Myomectomy

Having three children via C-section after undergoing a major surgery like a myomectomy is no small task. My journey to motherhood was not straightforward - it was marked by a series of challenges, triumphs, and intentional choices. Being proactive is essential. The myomectomy, though lifesaving, left me with scars and potential risk factors, particularly for future pregnancies. I knew that ensuring a smooth healing process along with reducing the risk of fibroid recurrence and preparing my body for childbirth required a holistic approach.

The Role of Diet

The foundation of my recovery and subsequent healthy pregnancies was my diet, nutrition, and lifestyle adjustments. I focused on nutrient-dense, anti-inflammatory foods (https://ninalemtirlifestylegroup.com/api/document/30_ Day_Anti_Inflammatory_Guidance_PlanTemplate)

I realised that what I put into my body would either hinder or help my healing, so I made the conscious decision to focus on nutrient-dense, anti-inflammatory foods that supported my body's ability to repair and thrive.

Nutrient-dense foods became the cornerstone of my meals. I prioritised leafy greens like kale, spinach, and huckle berry, which are rich in vitamins, minerals, and antioxidants. Cruciferous vegetables such as broccoli, cauliflower, and Brussels sprouts (in moderation) played a big role too, as they are known to support hormonal balance. I incorporated sweet potatoes and squash for their beta-carotene and other essential nutrients, and whole grains like quinoa and amaranth provided fiber and sustained energy.

To reduce inflammation, I leaned heavily on foods with natural anti-inflammatory properties. Fatty acids from sources like flaxseeds, chia seeds, and walnuts were a daily staple, as were avocados for their healthy monounsaturated fats. I used spices like turmeric, ginger, garlic, and celery for natural salts in my cooking to amplify the anti-inflammatory effects. These were not just ingredients; they were powerful tools in my healing journey.

I also embraced colourful fruits like berries, which are loaded with antioxidants that combat oxidative stress, and citrus fruits, which provided a steady dose of vitamin C. Even snacks became an opportunity to nourish my body, with choices like raw nuts, seeds, and hummus paired with sliced cucumbers or carrots.

Making these dietary changes was not always easy coming from being addicted to junk food, but it was a necessary part of reclaiming my health. Each meal became a deliberate act of self-care, and I saw the impact over time—not only in my recovery from surgery but also in my ability to carry three healthy pregnancies after years of challenges.

Through this journey, I learned that food is more than just fuel; it is medicine for the body and a foundation for healing and thriving that promote tissue repair and reduced the risk of adhesion formation. Incorporating foods rich in vitamins A, C, and E, along with zinc and omega-3 fatty acids, was essential for collagen synthesis and maintaining elasticity in my healing tissues. Having a morning and night time routine formed the foundation of my nutritional healing. I bio-hacked daily and avoided processed foods and anything that could contribute to inflammation or hinder my recovery. Instead, my meals became a celebration of healing—colourful, balanced, and thoughtfully chosen to nourish my body from the inside out.

When I say I "bio-hacked" daily, I mean I intentionally made small, strategic changes to optimise my body's healing processes. While the term "bio-hacking" might sound scientific or complex, it is really about using natural and accessible methods to support your body's ability to function at its best. For me, this meant eliminating processed foods, refined sugars, and anything that could trigger inflammation or slow down recovery.

As a result, my meals became fuel for healing —vibrant, balanced, and thoughtfully curated to nourish my body from the inside out. Think colourful salads bursting with raw vegetables, herbs, and seeds, or roasted root vegetables paired with whole grains like quinoa. I enjoyed the satisfied energised feeling after meals rather than the bloated and tired feeling I used to experience. Every bite I took was a step toward rebuilding my strength, ensuring my tissues healed effectively, and preventing complications like adhesions.

By prioritising nutrient-dense, anti-inflammatory foods and maintaining daily habits that supported my healing, I was able to regain control of my body and my health. These intentional choices were a powerful reminder that recovery is not just about medical procedures—it is about what you do every day to nurture your body and promote healing from within.

It is simply incorporating foods rich in vitamins A, C, and E, along with zinc and omega-3 fatty acids, was essential for collagen synthesis and maintaining elasticity in my healing tissues. These nutrients promote tissue repair and reduce the risk of adhesion formation, both of which were critical for my recovery. Foods like carrots, sweet potatoes, and spinach provided a wealth of vitamin A, while citrus fruits, bell peppers, and strawberries were my go-to sources for vitamin C. Almonds, sunflower seeds, green pumpkin seeds, and avocado delivered vitamin E, while walnuts, chia seeds, and flaxseeds supplied omega-3s to combat inflammation and support tissue healing.

Establishing a morning and nighttime routine became the foundation of my nutritional healing. These routines gave me structure and allowed me to remain consistent in my choices. In the morning, I would start my day with a nutrient-packed smoothie containing leafy greens, berries, flaxseeds, and plant-based protein and my supplements. At night, my meals were lighter but equally nourishing—often a bowl of vegetable and bean soup or a plate of steamed greens with a drizzle of olive oil and lemon.

Lifestyle Adjustments for Healing

Beyond food, I embraced a lifestyle that supported my body's natural healing processes. Gentle movement, such as walking and prenatal yoga, became my go-to. This helped improve circulation, preventing excessive scar tissue buildup and promoting flexibility in my abdominal area. I prioritised sleep and stress reduction activities like regular exercise, as I understood how crucial they were for my body's ability to repair itself. Practices like meditation and deep breathing exercises kept me grounded and calm, reducing the physiological effects of stress on my recovery and pregnancies.

Nutrition: The Unsung Hero

When it came to reclaiming my health, nutrition was not just a supporting player; it was the star of the show. I did not just eat to fill my stomach—I ate with intention, fueling my body with the nutrients it desperately needed to heal and thrive.

I discovered the power of targeted supplementation along the way, and let me tell you, it was a game-changer. My morning and night time routine became my secret weapon for rebuilding tissue and enhancing recovery. Plant-based protein powders were not just for gym-goers—they became my daily ally in strengthening my body from the inside out. High-performing probiotics were my ticket to a healthier gut, which I quickly learned was the foundation for everything from energy levels to hormone balance.

But it was not just about popping pills and powders. I sought out natural remedies like a detective on a mission, diving deep into what my body needed to support hormone balance and boost immunity. These were not quick fixes; they were pieces of a larger puzzle I was piecing together to create an internal environment that not only healed but thrived.

This journey was not easy—it took research, trial and error, and an unwavering commitment to listening to my body. As I watched my health transform, my energy return, and my dreams of healthy pregnancies become a reality, I realised that nutrition was not just a tool; it was my lifeline. It taught me to honour my body and give it what it needed to do what it was designed to do: heal, grow, and flourish.

Every intentional choice I made—what I ate, how I moved, and how I lived—helped me defy the odds and rewrite the script my doctors had handed me.

My diet and lifestyle did not just heal my body...they fortified it, transforming what once seemed impossible into a reality. Before adopting my new nutrition and wellness regimen, the thought of enduring one major surgery—let alone surviving three—felt like the end of my story. I was worn down; my body was struggling under the weight of years of neglect and untreated health issues.

But everything changed when I made the decision to take control of my health. Through intentional dietary choices and consistent lifestyle adjustments, I gave my body the tools it needed to not only recover, but also to thrive. My diet became a source of strength (anyone who knows me knows that when I get the "bit between my teeth" there is no letting go! lol), packed with foods that fueled my healing and resilience: leafy greens rich in vitamins, omega-3 fatty acids to combat inflammation, and nutrient-dense staples like quinoa, nuts, and berries to provide energy and repair damaged tissues. I would always keep some unsalted nuts in my handbag on the go.

This holistic approach fortified my body from the inside out. By addressing inflammation, improving circulation, and promoting cellular repair, I was able to rebuild my health in a way that prepared me for the physical demands of motherhood.

What once felt like the end of my story became the beginning of a new chapter. My fortified body carried life safely three times, even after the trauma of major surgery that could have left me with nothing but regret. My recovery was not just about healing—it was about exercising my power and proving that a diagnosis or a surgery does not define what is possible for your future.

Through my journey, I have learned that your body is capable of incredible things when you provide it with the right tools. My diet and lifestyle did not just save me—they became the foundation of the life I had dreamed of…a life that includes the joy of motherhood and the resilience to overcome any challenge.

By focusing on reducing adhesions and scar tissue, I avoided complications like uterine rupture or the excruciating pain so often linked to pregnancies which follow major surgeries. But the real testament to this journey was my second pregnancy with Vanea.

This time around, it felt almost unreal. I was so full of energy and strength that I wore heels until I was eight months pregnant. Heels! I was even hopping on and off flights, juggling life and work with ease, marveling at how effortless everything felt. It was such a stark contrast to what I had been through before that I had to pinch myself at times—I could not believe how different, how joyous, this pregnancy was.

These changes did not happen by accident. They were the result of relentless dedication, of learning to nourish my body and honour its needs. My journey is proof that when you give your body the right tools, it can do extraordinary things. It matters because this is not just my story—it is a blueprint for what is possible when you reclaim control over your health.

A Message for Women on Similar Journeys

This journey taught me that healing is possible, even after the most challenging surgeries. It is not just about medical interventions but also about how we show up for our bodies every day. For anyone facing similar obstacles, know that your diet, lifestyle, and mindset can be powerful tools in transforming your health and achieving your dreams of motherhood.

What is a Myomectomy?

"Myomectomy is the most adhesiogenic surgical procedure and postoperative adhesions can have a significant impact on the ability to conceive." (Mercorio et al., 2023)

It is a surgical procedure designed to remove uterine fibroids while preserving the uterus. For many women, this operation is a vital step toward reclaiming their health and well-being, especially when fibroids cause significant discomfort or complications. Unlike a hysterectomy, which involves the removal of the entire uterus, a myomectomy allows women to retain their reproductive capabilities, making it a popular choice for those wishing to conceive in the future. Understanding this procedure empowers women, especially professional and entrepreneurial women, to make informed decisions about their health.

Post-surgery, it is crucial to recognise that recovery is not solely about healing from the operation but also about taking proactive steps to prevent fibroid regrowth. Nutrition plays a pivotal role in this process and supports your personal contributing factors. A balanced diet rich in whole foods, daily synergistic antioxidants, and anti-inflammatory properties help to support the body during recovery particularly internally. Incorporating low sugar fruits, vegetables, lean organic proteins, and whole grains provide essential nutrients that promote healing and overall health. By focusing on nourishing the body, women will create a strong foundation for their long-term optimal wellness.

Maintaining a healthy diet before and after a myomectomy not only aids recovery but also helps balance hormones, which influence the growth of fibroids. For instance, including foods that support estrogen metabolism, such as cruciferous vegetables (in moderation) and healthy fats, are beneficial. Additionally, staying hydrated with consistent electrolytes and reducing processed foods, sugars, and unhealthy fats further enhance recovery. By adopting these dietary changes, women take charge of their health and reduce the risk of fibroid recurrence significantly.

In addition to nutrition, embracing a holistic approach to wellness is essential. This includes regular exercise, stress management techniques, and adequate sleep. Engaging in physical activity improves circulation, boosts mood, and enhances overall recovery. Mindfulness practices, such as yoga or meditation, also play a significant role in reducing stress, which has been linked to hormone imbalances and fibroid growth. By integrating these practices into their routine, women will cultivate a healthier lifestyle that supports their recovery and prevents future complications.

The journey after a myomectomy is one of empowerment and self-care. Women who prioritise their well-being through mindful nutrition and holistic practices can significantly reduce the likelihood of repeat surgeries. By embracing this opportunity to learn and grow, professional and entrepreneurial women can not only heal their bodies but also inspire others in their community. Taking charge of one's health is a powerful statement, and with the right tools and knowledge, a fibroid-free future is within reach.

The Importance of Post-Surgery Care

Post-surgery care is a crucial component of recovery, especially for women who have undergone a myomectomy. The journey does not end when you leave the operating room; rather, this is the beginning of a new chapter in your health and well-being. By focusing on post-surgery care, you empower yourself to not only heal effectively but also to prevent the recurrence of fibroids. Understanding the importance of this phase allows you to take charge of your recovery and shape a future free from the burden of fibroid-related health issues.

Nutrition plays an instrumental role in post-surgery care. After a myomectomy, your body requires specific nutrients to heal properly and regain strength. Emphasising a diet rich in antioxidants, vitamins, and minerals can significantly enhance your recovery process. Foods like leafy greens, berries, lean proteins, and healthy fats provide the building blocks your body needs to repair tissues and fight inflammation. By adopting a well-balanced nutrition plan tailored to your recovery, you not only support your healing journey but also lay the foundation for optimised long-term health.

Hydration is another vital aspect of post-surgery care that should not be overlooked. Drinking adequate amounts of water supports your body's natural healing processes, aids digestion, and helps flush out toxins. Consider incorporating herbal teas and broths into your routine to enhance hydration while also providing additional nutrients. Staying properly hydrated will boost your energy levels, improve your mood, and facilitate a smoother recovery, allowing you to return to your daily activities with renewed vigor.

In addition to nutrition and hydration, self-care practices are essential for your emotional and physical well-being post-surgery. Engaging in gentle activities such as walking, yoga, or stretching can improve circulation and promote healing without putting undue stress on your body. Mindfulness practices, such as meditation or deep breathing exercises, can help alleviate anxiety and enhance a positive mindset during your recovery. Prioritising self-care not only enhances your physical recovery but also nurtures your emotional resilience, empowering you to embrace this transformative period with confidence.

Lastly, embodying a supportive environment significantly impacts your post-surgery experience. Surrounding yourself with people who understand your journey and can offer encouragement and assistance is not just helpful—it is enriching.

I vividly recall my recovery. Right after surgery, I often felt physically and emotionally vulnerable. But what made all the difference was the unwavering support of my sister, who showed up daily to help with the small yet overwhelming tasks. Some as simply sitting with me when I felt low, or helping me to prepare meals. She reminded me to take my supplements, encouraged me to walk a little when I was ready, and even brought me fresh herbs and greens from the market to ensure I stayed on track with my nutrition plan. Her presence was a lifeline, grounding me in hope when doubt about the future threatened to creep in.

Then there was Sharon, one of the first women I coached. She had undergone a similar surgery but was struggling to balance her recovery with caring for her young children. Sharon felt isolated and overwhelmed, convinced she had to do everything herself. Through our sessions, we created a plan to involve her family and close friends in her healing journey. Her mother began preparing anti-inflammatory meals, her best friend organised a carpool to get her kids to school, and a neighbor helped with laundry. As Sharon was brave enough to ask for help and let go of the pressure to manage everything alone, she not only recovered faster but also felt more emotionally supported. This gave her the strength to focus on healing.

Alternatively, support can be sourced from individuals who have experienced similar situations, not just from close family or friends. When I joined an online support group for women recovering from fibroid surgery, I was amazed at the wealth of shared experiences and encouragement. One woman's story of overcoming complications and thriving afterward inspired me to see my own challenges as temporary rather than long term and overwhelming..

These case studies illustrate that the path to recovery need not be undertaken alone. When you allow others to support you, you create a space for healing that goes beyond the physical—it nurtures your spirit and fuels your resilience. Whether it is leaning on family, enlisting friends to help with practical tasks, or finding solidarity in a support group, a strong network turns what feels like an uphill climb into a shared and manageable experience.

Healing is not just about what happens to your body; it is also about the energy and encouragement you allow into your space. Surround yourself with people who lift you up, and you will find that the weight of recovery becomes lighter and more bearable.

CHAPTER 2

THE ROLE OF NUTRITION IN RECOVERY

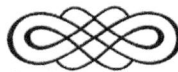

How Diet Affects Hormonal Balance

Diet plays a crucial role in maintaining hormonal balance, especially for women who have undergone a myomectomy. Hormones such as estrogen and progesterone significantly influence the growth of fibroids. A diet rich in whole foods, including fruits, vegetables, whole grains, and lean proteins, can help regulate these hormones, minimising the risk of fibroid regrowth. By focusing on nutrient-dense options, you empower your body to function optimally, supporting your recovery and overall health.

Incorporating healthy fats into your diet is essential for hormonal health. Omega-3 fatty acids, found in fish, flaxseeds, and walnuts, help reduce inflammation and promote balanced hormone levels. Additionally, these fats can support the production of hormones like progesterone, which counteracts the effects of estrogen. As you create your nutrition plan, prioritising sources of healthy fats plays a crucial role in establishing a more stable hormonal environment. This balance may significantly contribute to reducing the likelihood of fibroid recurrence.

Healthy fats are essential for hormone regulation, as they provide the building blocks for the production of hormones and help your body maintain equilibrium. Including these fats in your diet does not have to be complicated or expensive—there are plenty of accessible and nutrient-rich options to choose from.

Avocados, for instance, are a versatile source of healthy monounsaturated fats. Whether sliced into salads, blended into smoothies, or spread on whole-grain toast, they are an easy way to nourish your body. Nuts like almonds and walnuts are another fantastic option; a small handful as a snack or sprinkled over oatmeal can provide a satisfying dose of omega-3 fatty acids and vitamin E, both of which support hormonal health and reduce inflammation.

Seeds are another powerhouse addition to your diet. Flaxseeds, for example, are not only rich in omega-3s but also contain lignans, which have been shown to help balance estrogen levels. Sprinkle them over your morning porridge, blend them into smoothies, or mix them into plant-based yogurt. Similarly, chia seeds are great puddings or used as a topping for salads or soups.

Cold-pressed oils, such as extra virgin olive oil, are excellent sources of healthy fats. A drizzle of extra virgin olive oil over roasted vegetables or as part of a salad dressing provides antioxidants and promotes cardiovascular health while supporting hormone balance. For variety, I love to take 2 tablespoons of extra virgin olive oil in the morning.

If you enjoy smoothies, you can also incorporate plant-based sources of fats, such as almond milk, hemp seeds, or a small spoonful of nut butter. These not only enhance the taste and texture but also deliver the healthy fats your body needs.

By intentionally incorporating these accessible, nutrient-dense whole foods into your diet, you are not just nourishing your body—you are creating an environment that supports hormonal stability and reduces the risk of fibroid recurrence. The journey to healing and prevention starts with what is on your plate, and these simple, everyday choices can have a powerful impact over time.

Additionally, high-fibre foods help eliminate excess estrogen, promoting hormonal balance. Many everyday options make this simple to achieve. For fruits, try green apples, oranges, bananas, and berries. Common vegetables like carrots, broccoli, spinach, and sweet potatoes are easy to add to meals. Legumes such as lentils, chickpeas, and black beans are versatile and affordable, while whole grains like brown rice, organic oats, and whole-wheat bread are great for everyday use. These accessible choices support your body's natural detox processes, helping to reduce the risk of fibroid recurrence.

This is particularly vital for women with a history of fibroids since elevated estrogen levels can stimulate fibroid growth. Incorporating a variety of fibre-rich foods into your daily meals not only aids digestion but also supports your hormonal health, providing a proactive approach to preventing future complications.

Most importantly, hydration cannot be overlooked when discussing dietary impacts on hormonal balance. Drinking plenty of water helps flush out toxins and supports liver function, a key player in hormone metabolism. Herbal teas, such as green tea and spearmint, can be beneficial as well, offering antioxidants and compounds that may help regulate hormones. By prioritising hydration, you create a supportive internal environment for your body, enhancing your recovery process and reducing the risk of fibroid regrowth.

Finally, mindfulness in your eating habits is vital. Stress and emotional well-being significantly affect hormonal balance. Practicing mindful eating can reduce stress levels, leading to better hormonal regulation. Take the time to enjoy your meals, listen to your body's hunger cues, and appreciate the nourishment you provide. By adopting a holistic approach to your diet—one that encompasses nutrition, hydration, and mindfulness—you position yourself on a path toward lasting health and vitality, reducing the likelihood of facing repeat surgeries in the future.

Nutrients Essential for Healing

Nutrients play a pivotal role in the healing process, especially for women recovering from a myomectomy. After surgery, your body is in a delicate state, and providing it with the right nutrients can accelerate healing, minimise complications, and reduce the risk of fibroid regrowth. Embracing a diet rich in specific vitamins and minerals will not only support your recovery but also empower you to take control of your health and well-being.

Protein is one of the most crucial nutrients for healing. It serves as the building block for tissues and aids in the repair of damaged cells. Incorporating high-quality protein sources such as lean meats, fish, fortified organic foods, and legumes, into your daily meals can significantly enhance your body's ability to recover. These foods provide essential amino acids that are vital for the synthesis of new proteins, supporting your body's healing processes. Prioritising protein in your diet will help you regain strength and stamina as you transition back to your daily activities.

In addition to protein, vitamins and minerals play an integral role in post-surgery recovery. Vitamin C, for example, is essential for collagen formation, which is crucial for wound healing. Citrus fruits, strawberries, bell peppers, and broccoli are excellent sources of this vitamin. Similarly, zinc is vital for immune function and tissue repair, making foods like nuts, seeds, and whole grains important additions to your meals. By focusing on a colourful variety of fruits and vegetables, you not only boost your nutrient intake but also enhance your body's natural defenses against inflammation and infection.

Healthy fats are another key component of a post-myomectomy diet. Omega-3 fatty acids, found in fatty fish, flaxseeds, and walnuts, possess anti-inflammatory properties that can help soothe post-surgical inflammation and promote overall health. Including these healthy fats in your diet can also support hormone balance, which is essential for preventing fibroid regrowth. By consciously choosing nutritious fats, you empower your body to heal more effectively while also maintaining a balanced hormonal environment.

Finally, I cannot overstate the importance of hydration. Water plays a critical role in every bodily function, including digestion and nutrient absorption. Staying well-hydrated with essential electrolytes promotes optimal circulation, ensuring that all the healing nutrients you consume reach the tissues in need. Aim to drink plenty of water throughout the day, and consider herbal teas or broths that can also provide hydration along with additional nutrients. By making these dietary choices, you are not only nurturing your body during recovery but also setting a strong foundation for long-term health and a fibroid-free future.

The Connection Between Nutrition and Fibroid Prevention

Recent groundbreaking research by Al-Handy Research Labs in the United States has unveiled new insights into the critical relationship between nutrition and fibroid prevention, especially for women post-myomectomy. Their findings highlight the direct impact of dietary patterns on hormonal balance, inflammation, and fibroid regrowth, providing a scientific foundation for what many health practitioners have observed anecdotally for years.

A well-balanced diet is not just about overall health—it is a powerful tool to reduce the risk of fibroid recurrence. Al-Handy's studies show that diets rich in whole, plant-based foods can significantly lower the likelihood of fibroid regrowth by regulating estrogen levels and reducing systemic inflammation. This means that the choices you make at the table have the potential to support your long-term recovery and promote lasting wellness.

Fruits, vegetables, whole grains, and plant-based proteins are essential components of a fibroid-prevention diet. Specific foods like dark leafy greens, berries, and avocados are rich in antioxidants and phytonutrients that directly counteract inflammation and stabilise hormonal fluctuations. Al-Handy's research also revealed that healthy fats, such as those found in nuts, seeds, and olive oil, play a pivotal role in creating a hormonally balanced environment, further reducing the risk of fibroid regrowth (https://obgyn.uchicago.edu/research/al-hendy-laboratory)

Conversely, the research warns against the consumption of processed foods and sugars, which have been linked to increased estrogen levels and chronic inflammation—key drivers of fibroid development. By minimising these items and focusing on whole, unprocessed foods, you can proactively support your body's natural healing mechanisms.

Meal planning is another vital tool for success. Preparing nutrient-dense meals in advance not only ensures you stay on track but also minimises stress, which is another contributor to hormonal imbalance. Intentional eating is more than just a lifestyle; it is a commitment to your health and reduced fibroid dominance.

By embracing the wisdom of both science and nutrition, you are not just recovering—you are reclaiming control of your body and its potential. With each nourishing choice, you are building the foundation for a healthier, thriving life. Let the evidence empower you to take this journey with confidence and hope.

CHAPTER 3

CREATING YOUR PERSONALISED NUTRITION PLAN

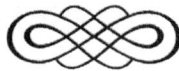

∞

Assessing Your Current Eating Habits

Assessing your current eating habits is an essential first step on your journey toward optimal health and well-being after a myomectomy. Many professional and entrepreneurial women lead busy lives, often prioritising work demands over personal health. Taking the time to evaluate your nutritional choices can empower you to make informed decisions that align with your recovery goals. By understanding your current eating patterns, you can identify areas for improvement and create a more balanced approach to nutrition that supports your unique needs.

Keep a detailed food diary for a week. Record all meals, snacks, and drinks. This exercise will provide valuable insights into your eating habits, helping you recognize patterns that may contribute to your overall health. Pay attention to the frequency of processed foods, sugar intake, and portion sizes. As you review your food diary, consider how your food choices make you feel physically and emotionally. This reflection will guide you in making adjustments that promote healing and vitality.

Next, evaluate the nutritional quality of your meals. Are you incorporating a variety of fruits, vegetables, whole grains, and lean proteins? A diverse colourful diet rich in essential nutrients significantly impacts your recovery journey positively. Focus on incorporating foods that support hormone balance and reduce inflammation, such as leafy greens, berries, nuts, and fatty fish. By consciously choosing nutrient-dense options, you empower yourself to create a foundation for a fibroid-free future while enjoying the pleasure of delicious and satisfying meals.

It is also important to assess your eating environment and habits. Are you eating while distracted, at your desk or in front of a screen? Mindful eating plays a crucial role in your overall relationship with food. Take the time to savour each bite, appreciating the textures and flavours of your meals. Creating a calm and inviting eating space can enhance your dining experience, allowing you to connect more deeply with your body's hunger and fullness cues. This practice not only fosters healthier relationships with food but also supports your body's healing process.

Finally, do not hesitate to seek support as you assess your eating habits. Consider working with a nutritionist or joining a community of women who share similar experiences. Surrounding yourself with individuals who understand your journey can provide encouragement and accountability. Remember, the path to recovery after a myomectomy is not just about physical healing; it is also about nurturing your mind and spirit. Embrace this opportunity to transform your eating habits and empower yourself to live a vibrant, fibroid-free life.

Setting Realistic Nutrition Goals

Setting realistic nutrition goals is a crucial step in the journey toward optimal recovery after a myomectomy. For professional and entrepreneurial women, balancing a busy lifestyle while prioritising health is significantly challenging. However, by establishing achievable nutrition goals, you can create a sustainable plan that supports healing and minimizes the risk of fibroid regrowth. Assessing your current habits and understanding where small adjustments can make a significant impact will empower you in your recovery journey.

Please see this resource that will help you empower your choices whilst shopping: https://ninalemtirlifestylegroup.com/api/document/Esse ntial_Health_Shopping_Guidance

Begin by evaluating your daily eating patterns and identifying areas that may need improvement. This could involve tracking your meals for a week to gain insight into your food choices and portion sizes. Rather than aiming for drastic changes, focus on one or two small adjustments at a time. For example, you might start by incorporating more fruits and vegetables into your meals or swapping out processed snacks for healthier options. These incremental changes are more manageable and can lead to lasting results, fostering a sense of accomplishment that motivates you to continue.

Next, consider setting specific and measurable goals that align with your lifestyle. Rather than vague aspirations like "eating healthier," aim for targets such as "adding an extra serving of vegetables to lunch three times a week." This specificity not only clarifies your objectives but also allows you to track your progress easily. Celebrate each milestone, no matter how small, as these victories build your confidence and reinforce your commitment to your health.

In addition to focusing on food choices, it is essential to consider the timing and frequency of your meals. Busy schedules often lead to irregular eating patterns, which may affect your recovery. Aim to establish a routine that includes balanced meals and snacks throughout the day. Setting a goal to eat every three to four hours should help maintain your energy levels and provide your body with the nutrients it needs for optimal healing. This structure not only supports your nutritional needs but also fits seamlessly into a professional lifestyle.

Finally, remember that nutrition is just one piece of the puzzle. Surround yourself with a supportive community, whether it is friends, family, or fellow women navigating similar experiences. Sharing your goals and progress with others provides motivation and accountability. As you work toward your nutrition goals, stay patient and compassionate with yourself. Healing is a process, and by setting realistic goals, you are taking empowered steps toward a fibroid-free future. Embrace this journey with confidence, knowing you are investing in your health and well-being.

Taylor, R.N., et al. "The Role of Inflammation in Uterine Fibroid Development." *Journal of Women's Health*, 2020.

Incorporating Anti-Inflammatory Foods

Incorporating anti-inflammatory foods into your diet is a strategic step in your journey toward recovery after a myomectomy. Understanding the role of inflammation in fibroid development is crucial. By embracing a diet rich in anti-inflammatory foods, you empower your body to heal and reduce the likelihood of fibroid regrowth. This approach not only supports physical health but also creates a sense of urgency over your well-being.

Start by including a variety of colourful fruits and vegetables in your meals. These nutrient-dense foods are packed with antioxidants, vitamins, and minerals that combat inflammation. Berries, leafy greens, and cruciferous vegetables such as broccoli and kale are particularly beneficial. They help to neutralise free radicals in the body and support overall cellular health. Experiment with vibrant salads or smoothies that incorporate these ingredients, making your meals as enjoyable as they are nourishing.

In addition to fruits and vegetables, healthy fats play a vital role in an anti-inflammatory diet. Incorporate sources of omega-3 fatty acids, such as fatty fish, walnuts, and flaxseeds, which have been shown to reduce inflammation. Extra virgin olive oil is another excellent choice, rich in mono-unsaturated fats and antioxidants. Use it as a base for salad dressings or as a finishing touch on roasted vegetables. These healthy fats not only enhance your diet but also contribute to a balanced, anti-inflammatory lifestyle that promotes recovery.

Whole grains should also be a cornerstone of your post-myomectomy nutrition plan. Opt for quinoa, brown rice, and oats, which provide fibre that supports digestive health and helps to stabilise blood sugar levels. These grains help you feel fuller longer, reducing the temptation to reach for processed foods that may contribute to inflammation. By prioritising whole grains, you create a foundation for sustained energy and overall well-being, essential for busy professional women like you.

Finally, I reiterate that you should not overlook the importance of hydration and herbal teas. Staying well-hydrated is essential for optimal bodily functions and can aid in reducing inflammation. Herbal teas, particularly those made from ginger and turmeric, can be excellent additions to your routine. They not only provide soothing warmth but also offer powerful anti-inflammatory properties. By consciously incorporating these elements into your daily life, you create a holistic approach to nutrition that promotes healing and empowers you in your fibroid-free journey.

CHAPTER 4

KEY FOOD GROUPS FOR
FIBROID-FREE LIVING

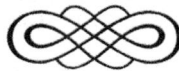

Fruits and Vegetables: Nature's Powerhouses

Fruits and vegetables are often hailed as nature's powerhouses, offering a wealth of nutrients essential for overall health and well-being. For professional and entrepreneurial women who have undergone a myomectomy, these vibrant foods can play a crucial role in recovery and prevention of fibroid regrowth. Packed with vitamins, minerals, antioxidants, and fibre, fruits and vegetables not only nourish the body but also support hormonal balance, which is vital for those looking to maintain their health after surgery.

Incorporating a colourful array of fruits and vegetables into your daily meals significantly enhance your nutritional profile. Leafy greens such as spinach and kale are rich in iron and folate, essential for recovery, while cruciferous vegetables like broccoli and cauliflower contain compounds that help regulate estrogen levels. This is particularly important for women concerned about fibroid recurrence. Maintaining hormonal balance is a key factor in preventing future growth. By making these foods a staple in your diet, you empower yourself with the tools needed to support your body's healing processes.

Moreover, fruits and vegetables are excellent sources of antioxidants, which combat oxidative stress and inflammation. Chronic inflammation has been linked to various health issues, including the development of fibroids. Berries, citrus fruits, and bell peppers are among the top choices for their high antioxidant content. Including these foods in your diet not only aids recovery but also promotes long-term health, allowing you to thrive both personally and professionally. Embracing these natural powerhouses can transform your meals into a celebration of health and vitality. (Balić, A., et al. "Oxidative Stress and Antioxidants in Uterine Fibroids: Pathophysiology and Clinical Implications." *ResearchGate*, 2023.)

Meal planning and preparation can be enjoyable and rewarding, especially when it involves colourful, nutrient-dense foods. Consider setting aside time each week to explore new recipes that highlight seasonal fruits and vegetables. Experimenting with different cooking methods, such as steaming, roasting, or blending into smoothies, can make healthy eating exciting and flavourful. By prioritising these foods in your life, you are not just nurturing your body but also setting a positive example for other women in your circle, inspiring them to take charge of their health journeys.

The journey towards fibroid-free living is a holistic one, where nutrition plays a central role. By embracing the power of fruits and vegetables, you are investing in your health and well-being. This commitment not only aids in recovery from myomectomy but also fosters a lifestyle that promotes balance and resilience. As you navigate your professional pursuits, remember that nourishing your body with nature's bounty equips you with the strength and energy to excel in all areas of life. You have the power to shape your future, and it starts with the choices you make today.

For detailed guidance on incorporating anti-inflammatory foods into your diet, refer to the **30-Day Anti-Inflammatory Guidance Plan** available at Nina Lemti Lifestyle Group.

https://ninalemtirlifestylegroup.com/api/document/3
0_Day_Anti_Inflammatory_Guidance_Plan

This resource provides practical tips and strategies to help you reduce inflammation, support healing, and promote long-term wellness.

Whole Grains: Fuel for Recovery

Whole grains serve as an essential component in the recovery journey post-myomectomy, acting as a powerful fuel source for healing and overall well-being. Rich in fibre, vitamins, and minerals, whole grains provide the nutrients necessary to support the body during recovery. Incorporating whole grains into your diet can significantly enhance your energy levels, stabilise blood sugar, and promote a healthy digestive system, all of which are crucial for women seeking to prevent the recurrence of fibroids.

When you choose whole grains over refined grains, you are making a conscious decision to nourish your body with higher-quality foods. Whole grains, such as quinoa, brown rice, oats, and whole wheat, retain their bran and germ, which are often stripped away in processed grains. This ensures that you receive the maximum benefits, including antioxidants and phytonutrients that support immune function. By focusing on whole grains, you are not only fueling your recovery but also empowering your body to fight against fibroid regrowth. ("Fibroids Diet," Healthline, https://www.healthline.com/health/fibroids-diet.)

Incorporating a variety of whole grains into your meals can be both delicious and satisfying. Start your day with a hearty bowl of oatmeal topped with fresh fruits and nuts, or enjoy a quinoa salad packed with colourful vegetables for lunch. Dinner can feature brown rice or farro as a base for a nutrient-dense stir-fry. The versatility of whole grains allows you to experiment with flavours and textures, making healthy eating an enjoyable part of your recovery process. Remember, every meal is an opportunity to nourish yourself and support your healing journey.

Moreover, whole grains contribute to sustained energy levels, which is particularly important for busy professional and entrepreneurial women. The fibre in whole grains helps regulate blood sugar, preventing the energy crashes that can lead to unhealthy snacking or poor food choices. By maintaining stable energy throughout the day, you will feel more focused and productive, allowing you to dedicate your time and efforts to your career and personal growth, all while prioritizing your health.

Lastly, it is essential to approach your recovery after major surgery with a positive mindset. Nourishing your body with whole grains can play a crucial role in physical healing while also fostering a sense of empowerment. By taking charge of your nutrition, you actively support your body's recovery process and promote overall well-being. As you explore the benefits of whole grains, remember that every small step towards a healthier diet is a meaningful stride towards long-term healing and resilience.

Healthy Fats: Supporting Hormonal Health

Healthy fats play a crucial role in supporting hormonal health, especially for women who are navigating the recovery process after a myomectomy. These beneficial fats are not just a source of energy; they are essential for the synthesis of hormones that regulate various bodily functions. For professional and entrepreneurial women, maintaining optimal hormonal balance is vital not only for physical health but also for mental clarity and productivity. By incorporating healthy fats into your diet, you can create a solid foundation for hormonal stability, helping to prevent the regrowth of fibroids.

One of the key components of healthy fats is omega-3 fatty acids, which are primarily found in fatty fish, flaxseeds, and walnuts. These fats have anti-inflammatory properties that can help reduce the inflammation often linked to fibroid growth. By actively including sources of omega-3s in your meals, you not only support your hormonal health but also promote overall wellness. Simple adjustments, such as adding salmon to your weekly menu or sprinkling flaxseeds on your morning yogurt, can make a significant difference in how you feel during your recovery.

Monounsaturated fats, found in foods like avocados, olive oil, and nuts, also play a vital role in hormonal balance. These fats help to stabilise insulin levels, which is crucial for maintaining healthy reproductive hormones. For busy women managing careers and personal lives, incorporating these fats can be both easy and delicious. A quick salad drizzled with olive oil or a slice of avocado on whole-grain toast can provide the nourishment your body needs without requiring extensive meal prep. Embracing these fats will support your hormonal health and enhance your overall energy levels.

In addition to omega-3s and monounsaturated fats, it is important not to overlook the significance of saturated fats from high-quality sources like grass-fed meats and coconut oil. While often misunderstood, these fats contribute to hormone production when consumed in moderation. They can provide the building blocks necessary for hormone synthesis, particularly for women recovering (Healthline.com/nutrition/balance-hormones) from surgical procedures like myomectomy. By choosing the right sources of saturated fats, you can ensure that your body has the nutrients it needs to thrive.

Finally, remember that the journey to hormonal balance is a holistic one. Pairing healthy fats with a diverse range of nutrient-dense foods, including fruits, vegetables, and whole grains, will amplify their benefits. As you recover from your myomectomy, focus on nourishing your body with the right fats while staying mindful of how they fit into your overall dietary plan. This balanced approach will empower you to take control of your health, helping to prevent the regrowth of fibroids and supporting a vibrant, energetic life. Embrace the power of healthy fats and watch as they contribute to your journey towards wellness and success.

Proteins: Building Blocks for Healing

Proteins are fundamental to the body's healing process, especially for women recovering from a myomectomy. After surgery, your body requires essential nutrients to repair tissues, regenerate cells, and restore overall health. Proteins, often referred to as the building blocks of life, are crucial in this context. By incorporating the right proteins into your diet, you can enhance your healing journey and give your body the tools it needs to regain strength and vitality.

In my recovery, I discovered that the quality of protein mattered just as much as the quantity. I removed red meat and poor-quality proteins, such as highly processed meats like sausages, hot dogs, and deli meats, from my diet, as they contribute to inflammation and hormonal imbalances. These processed options often contain preservatives, additives, and unhealthy saturated fats that research suggests have been identified as endocrine-disrupting chemicals (EDCs) that can disrupt your body's natural hormonal rhythms. Instead, I focused on cleaner, nutrient-rich organic protein sources that supported healing and balanced my hormones. Instead, I focused on lean organic proteins, fish, legumes, fortified plant-based products, and seeds. These high-quality protein sources provided the essential amino acids my body needed to repair itself, while also promoting hormonal balance—a key factor in preventing fibroid regrowth.

Beyond physical healing, protein was a lifeline for maintaining energy and supporting my immune system. After surgery, hormonal fluctuations, and the physical toll of recovery left me feeling drained. By prioritising protein-rich meals, I found a steady source of energy that stabilised my blood sugar levels and prevented the cravings that often lead to unhealthy choices. This stability was essential not just for my recovery but for building long-term resilience.

Proteins also played a surprising role in my emotional recovery. Healing is not just physical—it is mental and emotional, too. Amino acids found in proteins are critical for producing neurotransmitters that regulate mood and cognitive function. A nutrient-rich, protein-focused diet gave me the mental clarity and emotional strength to navigate the challenges of post-surgery life with confidence.

As you navigate your own healing journey, remember that nutrition is a powerful ally. By consciously choosing high-quality proteins and avoiding inflammatory foods, you are giving your body the best chance to heal and thrive. Your dietary choices do not just support recovery—they lay the foundation for a vibrant, fibroid-free future. Trust in your body's ability to heal and honour it with the nutrition it needs to flourish beyond surgery.

CHAPTER 5

MEAL PLANNING AND PREPARATION

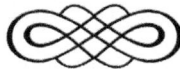

Crafting a Weekly Meal Plan

Crafting a weekly meal plan is an empowering step toward reclaiming your health after a myomectomy. As a professional woman, your time is valuable, and organising your meals can save you both time and energy throughout the week. A thoughtfully designed meal plan not only helps you avoid the stress of last-minute decisions but also ensures that you are nourishing your body with the right nutrients to support recovery and prevent fibroid regrowth. By taking control of your meals, you create a foundation for a healthier lifestyle.

Begin by assessing your nutritional needs based on your specific recovery goals. Incorporate foods rich in fibre, antioxidants, and healthy fats, which can help reduce inflammation and support hormonal balance. Make a list of your favourite meals and snacks that align with these nutritional principles. Consider integrating a variety of colourful fruits and vegetables, whole grains, lean organic proteins, and healthy fats into your meals. This diversity not only enhances the nutritional value of your diet but also makes your meals more appealing and satisfying.

Next, dedicate some time to planning your meals for the week. Choose a day when you can focus on this task without distractions. Start by selecting recipes that can be prepared in bulk or can be easily modified for different meals. For example, a roasted vegetable mix can serve as a side dish, a salad base, or be blended into a soup. Aim for a balance of flavours and textures to keep your meals exciting. Once you have chosen your recipes, create a grocery list that includes all the ingredients you will need, ensuring you have everything on hand to minimise the temptation of unhealthy last-minute choices.

Once your meals are planned and your groceries are purchased, consider meal prepping as an essential part of your strategy. Set aside a few hours on the weekend to prepare your meals in advance. Cook larger portions of grains and proteins, chop vegetables, and assemble salads that can be stored in the refrigerator. This preparation allows you to simply grab and go during busy weekdays, making it easier to stick to your plan. Remember, the effort you put into meal prep not only saves you time but also reinforces your commitment to your health and well-being.

Lastly, be flexible and kind to yourself as you navigate this new routine. Life can be unpredictable, and there will be days when you may not stick to your plan perfectly. Embrace those moments and view them as opportunities to learn and adapt. Remember to always focus on what your next empowering action step will be. If you find a meal that you love or a new recipe that excites you, feel free to swap it in for the following week. The goal is to create a sustainable and enjoyable eating pattern that supports your recovery and prevents fibroid regrowth, empowering you to lead a vibrant and fulfilling life.

Smart Grocery Shopping Tips

Smart grocery shopping is essential for professional and entrepreneurial women who are navigating the journey of post-myomectomy recovery. Understanding how to stock your kitchen with nourishing foods empowers you to take charge of your health and support your body's healing process. Begin by crafting a thoughtful grocery list that prioritises whole, nutrient-dense foods. Focus on fruits, vegetables, whole grains, lean organic proteins, and healthy fats. This list will serve as your roadmap, ensuring that you have the right ingredients at your fingertips to create meals that promote wellness and prevent fibroid regrowth. Utilise auto ship for your essential items so you do not have to go looking for those foundational items (saves time and resources).

When you arrive at the grocery store, consider exploring the perimeter first, where fresh produce, meats, and dairy items are typically located. This area is often where you will find the healthiest options, far removed from processed foods that hinder your recovery. As you browse through the colourful array of fruits and vegetables, aim to select organic options whenever possible, as they are free from harmful pesticides and chemicals. Filling your cart with vibrant produce not only enhances your meals but also provides your body with essential vitamins and minerals that support healing.

Seasonal shopping is another smart strategy to enhance both your nutrition and your budget. By choosing fruits and vegetables that are in season, you can enjoy their peak flavour and nutritional value while saving money. Seasonal items are often fresher, which means they contain more nutrients. Take the time to learn which foods are in season throughout the year and incorporate them into your meal plans. This practice not only diversifies your diet but also connects you to the natural rhythms of food, emphasising a deeper appreciation for the nourishment you provide to your body.

In addition to focusing on fresh produce, do not overlook the importance of healthy proteins and whole grains. Incorporate a variety of organic lean proteins, such as fish, beans, and legumes, to support muscle repair and overall health. Whole grains like quinoa, brown rice, and oats offer fibre that aids in digestion and helps maintain stable blood sugar levels. Stocking your pantry with these staples ensures you always have the foundation for a wholesome meal. By making conscious choices while grocery shopping, you set yourself up for success in your recovery journey.

Finally, remember to practice mindful shopping by avoiding impulse buys and processed snacks that can undermine your health goals. Take a moment to read labels and familiarise yourself with ingredients that may not align with your nutritional needs. Establishing a habit of mindful grocery shopping allows you to cultivate healthier choices every day. With a proactive approach and a commitment to nourishing your body, you should thrive in your post-myomectomy recovery and progress towards a fibroid-free future.

Simple, Nutritious Recipes for Busy Women

Eating well is essential for women recovering from a myomectomy, especially for busy professionals and entrepreneurs who juggle multiple responsibilities. Simple, nutritious recipes will empower you to nourish your body without adding stress to your already packed schedule. The key is to embrace meals that are easy to prepare, packed with essential nutrients, leading to the prevention of fibroid regrowth. By prioritising nutrition, you not only support your healing journey but also maintain the energy needed to thrive in your professional life.

One simple recipe to consider is a quinoa bowl loaded with colourful vegetables. Start with cooked quinoa as your base, which is rich in protein and fibre. Add sautéed red onions, spinach, bell peppers, and broccoli for a boost of vitamins and minerals. Top it off with a sprinkle of sunflower seeds and a drizzle of extra virgin olive oil for healthy fats. This dish is not only easy to prepare but can also be made in advance and stored in the refrigerator for quick lunches or dinners throughout the week. Each bite offers a blend of nutrients that promote healing and keeps you feeling satisfied.

Another time-saving option is a smoothie packed with antioxidants and fibre. Blend together a banana, a handful of spinach, a scoop of high quality protein powder, and a cup of almond milk (or your preference). For added nutrition, toss in some chia seeds or flaxseeds, which are excellent sources of omega-3 fatty acids. Smoothies are incredibly versatile and can be customised based on your preferences. Preparing them in the morning or even the night before will help you start your day energised, all while ensuring you get the nutrients necessary for recovery.

For a heartier choice, consider making a one-pan baked wild salmon with sweet potatoes and asparagus. Simply season the wild salmon with lemon, garlic, and herbs, then arrange it alongside chopped sweet potatoes and asparagus on a baking sheet. This meal is rich in omega-3 fatty acids and vitamins A and C, supporting your overall health. The best part is that it cooks in about 30 minutes, allowing you to enjoy a delicious, balanced meal without spending hours in the kitchen.

Lastly, do not overlook the power of homemade soups. A hearty lentil soup can be made in bulk and frozen for easy access. Combine lentils with diced tomatoes, carrots, celery, and spices for flavour. Lentils are high in protein and fibre, helping to regulate blood sugar levels and keep you feeling full longer. Simply reheat a portion when you are short on time, and you have a warm, nutritious meal that aligns perfectly with your health goals. Remember, investing in your nutrition is a powerful step towards living fibroid-free, and these simple recipes are your allies in this journey.

CHAPTER 6

SUPPLEMENTS AND HERBAL REMEDIES

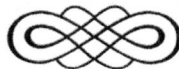

Understanding the Role of Supplements

As a Nutrition Lifestyle Strategist, I specialise in helping women optimise their healing and achieve faster, longer-lasting results by leveraging the power of nutrition and lifestyle. Understanding the role of supplements in your post-myomectomy recovery is a crucial step toward maintaining your health and preventing the regrowth of fibroids. For professional and entrepreneurial women like you, taking charge of your wellness means making informed decisions that align with your goals and busy lives. Supplements, when combined with a balanced diet, provide essential nutrients to support your body's healing, hormonal balance, and overall resilience.

Vitamins and minerals are the foundation of well-being. Vitamin D, for instance, is not only vital for calcium absorption and bone health but also plays a role in regulating immune function and cell growth. Many women, especially those juggling demanding careers and limited sun exposure, are deficient in vitamin D. Magnesium is another key player, aiding in hormonal balance, reducing muscle tension, and promoting relaxation. Incorporating these nutrients into your supplement routine can significantly support your recovery while minimising the risk of fibroid regrowth.

Herbal supplements also bring transformative benefits. Herbs like chaste tree berry (Vitex) and green tea extract are known for their ability to support hormonal equilibrium and reduce the likelihood of fibroid redevelopment. Anti-inflammatory powerhouses like turmeric and ginger can help your body heal more efficiently by reducing inflammation. As always, consult with a healthcare professional to ensure these choices suit your unique health profile and do not interfere with any medications.

Equally important are probiotics, which bolster your gut health—a critical factor in recovery and hormonal regulation. Surgery can disrupt your digestive system, making it essential to restore balance with high-quality probiotics. A healthy gut microbiome not only enhances nutrient absorption and immune support but also emphasises the hormonal harmony needed to sustain your recovery and long-term health.

Supplementation is not a one-size-fits-all solution; it is a personalised journey. As a Nutrition Lifestyle Strategist, I work closely with women to create customised supplementation plans tailored to their individual health histories and goals. By integrating the right supplements into your daily routine, you are investing in a fibroid-free future and building the foundation for a vibrant, fulfilling life. Every intentional step brings you closer to lasting health and freedom beyond surgery.

Herbal Allies for Hormonal Balance

Herbal allies play a pivotal role in supporting hormonal balance, especially for women navigating the challenges of post-myomectomy recovery. Many women who have undergone myomectomy struggle with hormonal fluctuations, which can lead to discomfort and even the potential for fibroid regrowth. Incorporating specific herbs into daily routines can serve as a natural and empowering approach to managing these issues. By understanding the properties of these herbal allies, women can take proactive steps toward reclaiming their health and well-being.

One of the most celebrated herbs for hormonal harmony is Vitex, also known as chaste tree. This herb has been used for centuries to help regulate menstrual cycles and alleviate symptoms of premenstrual syndrome. Vitex works by influencing the pituitary gland, which plays a key role in hormone production. For women recovering from myomectomy, balancing estrogen and progesterone levels is crucial. Regular use of Vitex can help restore this balance, promoting a more regulated cycle and reducing the risk of fibroid regrowth.

Another powerful herb to consider is Dong Quai, often referred to as the "female ginseng." This traditional Chinese herb is renowned for its ability to nourish and support the female reproductive system. Dong Quai can help improve blood circulation and regulate menstrual flow, making it an excellent choice for women experiencing hormonal imbalances post-surgery. Incorporating Dong Quai into herbal teas or supplements can provide a comforting way to support hormonal health while promoting overall vitality.

Maca root is another fantastic ally in the journey toward hormonal balance. Known for its adaptogenic properties, Maca can help the body adapt to stress while balancing energy levels and improving mood. This is particularly beneficial for women who may feel overwhelmed during their recovery. Rich in nutrients and minerals, Maca supports adrenal health, which in turn can help regulate hormone production. Including Maca in smoothies or as a supplement can offer a nourishing boost during this transformative time.

Finally, incorporating a variety of herbal teas, such as red clover or nettle, can provide additional support for hormonal balance. These herbs are rich in essential nutrients and can help detoxify the body, further supporting recovery. Drinking herbal teas regularly not only hydrates the body but also offers a moment of self-care and mindfulness. As women embrace these herbal allies, they empower themselves with knowledge and tools that enhance their recovery journey, paving the way for a healthier, fibroid-free future.

Consulting with Healthcare Professionals

Consulting with healthcare professionals is a pivotal step in your journey to a fibroid-free life after a myomectomy. As a professional or entrepreneurial woman, you understand the importance of making informed decisions, particularly when it comes to your health. Engaging with a team of healthcare providers allows you to access specialised knowledge that can significantly enhance your recovery process. By collaborating with gynecologists, nutritionists, and other health experts, you can create a comprehensive plan tailored to your unique needs, ensuring that you are well-equipped to prevent the regrowth of fibroids.

When you consult with your gynecologist, you gain valuable insights into the medical aspects of your recovery. They can provide you with essential information about your condition and help you understand the factors that may contribute to fibroid recurrence. This knowledge empowers you to take proactive steps in your health journey. Open communication with your doctor fosters a partnership where you can express your concerns and preferences, resulting in a tailored approach that aligns with your lifestyle and professional commitments.

In addition to gynecological care, working with a registered dietitian or nutritionist is crucial for developing a diet plan that supports your recovery. Nutrition plays a significant role in managing your overall health and preventing fibroid regrowth. A nutrition expert can guide you in making dietary choices that promote hormone balance, reduce inflammation, and enhance your body's natural healing processes. This collaboration not only provides you with a practical roadmap for eating but also instills confidence in your ability to influence your health positively.

Furthermore, consider consulting complementary healthcare professionals such as acupuncturists or herbalists. These practitioners can offer holistic approaches that work in conjunction with traditional medical care. Integrating alternative therapies can enhance your recovery by addressing stress levels, emotional well-being, and overall balance in your life. Exploring these options may introduce you to new methods of self-care that resonate with your values as a professional woman, enriching your journey toward wellness.

As you embrace the support of healthcare professionals, remember that you are not alone on this path. Each consultation, each conversation, and each dietary adjustment brings you closer to a healthier, fibroid-free life. By prioritising your health and seeking expert guidance, you demonstrate strength and determination. This proactive approach will not only benefit your recovery but also empower you to thrive in your personal and professional life, setting an inspiring example for other women in similar situations.

CHAPTER 7

LIFESTYLE CHANGES FOR LONG-TERM SUCCESS

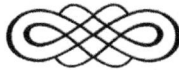

The Importance of Regular Exercise

Regular exercise is an essential component of a healthy lifestyle, particularly for women who have undergone a myomectomy. Engaging in physical activity not only aids in physical recovery but also plays a crucial role in maintaining overall well-being. For professional and entrepreneurial women, balancing the demands of work and personal life can be challenging, but prioritising exercise is a powerful step towards enhancing your health and preventing the recurrence of fibroids. By incorporating regular movement into your routine, you empower yourself to take control of your health journey.

Exercise can significantly improve circulation, which is vital for healing and recovery after surgery. Improved blood flow helps deliver essential nutrients to the tissues that need it most, promoting faster healing and reducing inflammation. For women recovering from a myomectomy, this means a more efficient body able to repair itself and maintain optimal function. Furthermore, physical activity helps to strengthen the pelvic floor muscles, which can support reproductive health and reduce the risk of complications. By committing to regular exercise, you set the stage for a smoother recovery and a more resilient body.

In addition to physical benefits, regular exercise also plays a crucial role in mental health. The demands of professional life can often lead to stress, anxiety, and feelings of being overwhelmed. Exercise releases endorphins, the body's natural mood lifters, which can help combat stress and promote a sense of well-being. For women navigating post-surgery recovery, this emotional boost is invaluable. It not only aids in coping with the physical challenges but also enhances motivation and focus, enabling you to tackle your professional responsibilities with renewed vigour.

Incorporating exercise into your daily routine does not have to be a daunting task. Finding activities you enjoy can make a significant difference in your commitment to staying active. Whether it is brisk walking, yoga, swimming, or dancing, the key is to choose movements that resonate with you personally. As a busy professional woman, consider scheduling your workouts just as you would any important meeting. This approach transforms exercise from a chore into a non-negotiable part of your life, reinforcing the message that your health is a priority.

Invariably, regular exercise is a powerful tool in your arsenal for preventing fibroid regrowth and enhancing your overall quality of life. By embracing a physically active lifestyle, you not only support your body's recovery but also cultivate resilience, mental clarity, and emotional stability. Remember, you are not just investing in your health; you are setting a powerful example for others. As you move forward on your journey, let every step you take be a testament to your commitment to a fibroid-free life, empowered by the strength that comes from regular exercise.

Stress Management Techniques

Stress management is a crucial component of recovery and overall well-being, especially for professional women navigating the challenges of fibroid management post-myomectomy. Understanding that stress can exacerbate physical symptoms and influence hormonal balance is the first step toward mastering effective techniques. Incorporating stress management practices into daily routines not only supports emotional health but also enhances the body's ability to heal. By prioritising self-care, women can create a nurturing environment that fosters recovery and prevents the recurrence of fibroids.

One effective technique for managing stress is mindfulness meditation. This practice encourages individuals to focus on the present moment and become aware of their thoughts and feelings without judgment. For professional women, dedicating just a few minutes each day to mindfulness can significantly reduce anxiety and promote a sense of calm. Setting aside this time helps to create mental space, allowing for clearer thinking and improved decision-making. As you cultivate mindfulness, you may find that it enhances your overall resilience, making it easier to handle the pressures of both work and personal life.

Physical activity is another powerful stress reliever that can be easily integrated into a busy lifestyle. Engaging in regular exercise, whether it is a brisk walk, yoga session, or dance class, not only boosts endorphins but also improves overall physical health. Exercise helps in maintaining a healthy weight, which is essential for hormonal balance. For women recovering from myomectomy, finding enjoyable ways to move can transform stress into energy, allowing for a more positive outlook on life. Consider scheduling exercise sessions like appointments, making them a non-negotiable part of your day.

Nutrition plays a pivotal role in stress management as well. A well-balanced diet rich in whole foods, including fruits, vegetables, lean proteins, and healthy fats, provides the nutrients necessary for optimal brain function and mood stabilisation. Foods high in antioxidants, omega-3 fatty acids, and vitamins can be particularly helpful in combating stress. Implementing a nutrition plan that focuses on these elements not only supports recovery from surgery but also empowers women to take charge of their health and prevent the regrowth of fibroids. Meal prepping and planning can also reduce the stress of last-minute cooking decisions.

Finally, building a supportive network is vital to effective stress management. Engaging with friends, family, or support groups can provide a sense of belonging and understanding. Sharing experiences with others who have faced similar challenges can be incredibly empowering. Professional women should prioritise creating connections that offer emotional support and encouragement during recovery. Whether it is through organised meet-ups or online forums, having a community can significantly alleviate feelings of isolation, making the journey toward fibroid-free living much more manageable and uplifting.

Building a Support Network

Building a strong support network is essential for professional and entrepreneurial women navigating the journey of recovery after a myomectomy. This journey can feel overwhelming at times, but surrounding yourself with the right people can make all the difference. Your support network should include family, friends, healthcare professionals, and peers who understand the unique challenges you face. They can provide not only emotional support but also practical advice on nutrition and lifestyle choices that promote healing and prevent fibroid regrowth.

Start by reaching out to those closest to you. Share your experiences and goals with family and friends who can offer encouragement and understanding. They can become your cheerleaders, celebrating your successes, and helping you stay accountable to your nutrition and wellness plans. Consider organising regular check-ins, whether in person or virtually, to create a space where you can share challenges and triumphs related to your recovery journey. This connection can foster motivation and resilience, reminding you that you are not alone in this process.

In addition to your personal circle, seek out healthcare professionals who specialize in nutrition and women's health. A dietitian familiar with post-myomectomy recovery can provide tailored guidance and meal plans that support your specific needs. They can help you understand which foods promote healing, reduce inflammation, and prevent fibroid regrowth. Establishing a relationship with a healthcare provider who understands your situation will empower you to make informed choices about your nutrition and overall health.

Networking with other women who have undergone similar experiences can also be incredibly beneficial. Look for support groups, either online or in your local community, where you can connect with others who understand the physical and emotional challenges of recovery. Sharing stories and strategies can provide valuable insights and foster a sense of camaraderie. These connections will remind you that you are part of a larger community of women united in the pursuit of health and well-being.

Finally, do not underestimate the power of professional networks. Engage with organisations and forums that focus on women's health, entrepreneurship, and holistic wellness. These platforms can offer resources, workshops, and events that not only expand your knowledge but also help you connect with like-minded individuals. By actively participating in these communities, you can build a robust support network that empowers you to thrive in your personal and professional life, all while prioritizing your health and well-being.

CHAPTER 8

Empowering Yourself Through Knowledge

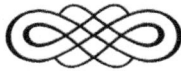

Staying Informed About Your Health

Staying informed about your health is crucial, especially after undergoing a myomectomy. As a professional or entrepreneurial woman, juggling various responsibilities can make it challenging to prioritise your well-being. However, understanding your body and its needs will empower you to make informed decisions that promote healing and prevent the recurrence of fibroids. Knowledge is the precursor to experience; it enables you to navigate your health journey with confidence and purpose.

One essential aspect of staying informed is recognising the importance of nutrition in your recovery. A well-balanced diet rich in whole foods, healthy fats, and lean proteins can significantly impact your recovery process and long-term health. Incorporating foods high in fibre, such as fruits, vegetables, and whole grains, can aid digestion and help maintain a healthy weight, which is pivotal in preventing fibroid regrowth. Educating yourself about which foods support hormonal balance can also enhance your overall well-being, making you feel more energised and focused in your personal and professional life.

Regular check-ups with your healthcare provider are another vital component of staying informed. These appointments provide an excellent opportunity to discuss your recovery progress, ask questions, and address any concerns you may have. Staying proactive in your healthcare allows you to catch any potential issues early and adapt your nutrition and lifestyle choices accordingly. Building a strong relationship with your healthcare team can empower you to advocate for your health and ensure you are receiving the best care possible.

In addition to medical appointments, utilising online resources and community support can enhance your knowledge. Joining forums or groups focused on women's health, especially those tailored to post-myomectomy recovery, can provide valuable insights and shared experiences. Learning from others who are on similar journeys can offer encouragement and practical tips for maintaining a healthy lifestyle. Engaging with expert blogs, podcasts, and webinars can further enrich your understanding of nutrition's role in preventing fibroid regrowth.

Lastly, remember that staying informed is an ongoing process. As new research emerges, being adaptable and willing to learn will serve you well in your health journey. Take the time to reflect on your experiences and continually seek out information that resonates with your unique situation. By prioritising your health education, you not only enhance your recovery but also equip yourself with the tools to thrive as a professional woman, ready to conquer the challenges ahead. Embrace this journey with optimism and determination, knowing that every step you take is a step towards a fibroid-free future.

Recognising Early Signs of Fibroid Regrowth

Recognising the early signs of fibroid regrowth is crucial for women who have undergone a myomectomy and are committed to maintaining their health and well-being. Knowledge is power, and by understanding the indicators of fibroid regrowth, you can take proactive steps to address any concerns. Common signs may include changes in menstrual patterns, such as increased heaviness or prolonged bleeding, which can signal the need for a closer look. Staying attuned to your body and noting any unusual symptoms can empower you to act quickly and consult with your healthcare provider.

Another important aspect to consider is the physical discomfort that may accompany fibroid regrowth. Many women report experiencing pelvic pain or pressure, which can be a sign that it is time to reassess your health strategies. It is essential to differentiate between typical post-surgical discomfort and new symptoms that warrant attention. Keep a journal to track any changes in your body, as this can be an invaluable tool when discussing your health with medical professionals. Remember, being proactive about your health is a key part of your journey toward fibroid-free living.

In addition to physical symptoms, emotional well-being plays a significant role in recognising fibroid regrowth. Stress and anxiety can manifest in various ways, including changes in your overall health. Take note of any shifts in your mood or energy levels, as these can be reflective of underlying issues. Surrounding yourself with a supportive community and engaging in stress-reducing activities such as yoga or meditation can enhance your emotional resilience. By prioritising your mental health, you are better equipped to face any health challenges that may arise.

Diet and nutrition are powerful allies in preventing fibroid regrowth, and being mindful of your eating habits is essential. Certain foods can promote hormonal balance and reduce inflammation, which are key factors in maintaining a healthy environment in your body. Incorporate plenty of fruits, vegetables, whole grains, and lean proteins into your meals. By fueling your body with nutrient-dense foods, you can help mitigate the risk of fibroid regrowth and support your overall health. Empower yourself through informed dietary choices that align with your recovery and long-term wellness goals.

Finally, never underestimate the importance of regular check-ups and open communication with your healthcare provider. Regular screenings can help identify any issues before they become significant concerns. Sharing your observations about your body and any symptoms you experience allows your medical team to provide tailored advice and support. Stay informed, stay proactive, and remember that you are not alone in this journey. Together, with the right knowledge and resources, you can navigate your path toward a fibroid-free life and thrive in your personal and professional endeavors.

Advocating for Your Health Needs

In your journey towards optimal health post-myomectomy, advocating for your health needs is a crucial step that empowers you to take control of your well-being. As professional and entrepreneurial women, you often juggle multiple responsibilities, making it easy to overlook your personal health. However, prioritising your health is not just beneficial for you; it also enables you to perform at your best in your career and personal life. By becoming your own health advocate, you foster a proactive approach to recovery and well-being that aligns with your ambitions and goals.

Start by educating yourself about your condition and the implications of a myomectomy. Understand the potential for fibroid regrowth and the lifestyle changes that can help mitigate this risk. Knowledge is power, and by being well-informed, you can engage in meaningful conversations with healthcare providers. Prepare questions in advance, seek clarity on treatment options, and discuss tailored nutrition and diet plans that support your recovery. This proactive stance not only enhances your understanding but also positions you as an active participant in your health journey.

Incorporate holistic practices into your routine that support both your physical and mental health. Nutrition plays a pivotal role in preventing fibroid regrowth, so focus on a balanced diet rich in whole foods, antioxidants, and anti-inflammatory ingredients. Collaborate with a nutritionist who specialised in post-myomectomy recovery to create a personalised meal plan that fuels your body and promotes healing. By making informed choices about what you eat, you are not just nurturing your body; you are sending a powerful message to yourself that your health is worth the investment.

Embrace the importance of community support in your advocacy efforts. Surround yourself with like-minded women who understand the challenges and triumphs of navigating life after a myomectomy. Joining support groups or online forums can provide you with valuable insights and encouragement. Sharing experiences, successes, and strategies can be incredibly empowering, reminding you that you are not alone in this journey. Together, you can hold each other accountable and celebrate milestones, reinforcing a collective commitment to health and wellness.

Lastly, remember that self-advocacy extends beyond medical appointments and dietary choices; it encompasses your overall lifestyle. Prioritise self-care and stress management techniques that resonate with you, whether it is meditation, yoga, or engaging in hobbies that bring you joy. By nurturing your mental and emotional health, you create a robust foundation for your physical recovery. Your journey towards fibroid-free living is uniquely yours, and by advocating for your health needs, you empower yourself to thrive in every aspect of your life, embracing a future filled with vitality and purpose.

CHAPTER 9

SUCCESS STORIES AND TESTIMONIALS

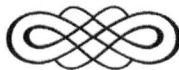

⌘

Inspiring Journeys of Recovery

Every woman's journey through recovery after a myomectomy is unique, yet many share similar experiences of resilience and hope. These inspiring stories highlight the strength and determination of women who have faced the challenges of fibroid surgery and emerged empowered, ready to reclaim their health and well-being. By embracing nutrition and making informed lifestyle choices, they have transformed their lives and created a future free from the fear of fibroid regrowth.

Consider the story of Maria, a successful entrepreneur who found herself sidelined by the physical and emotional toll of fibroids. After her myomectomy, Maria recognised the importance of nutrition in her healing process. She began to explore plant-based diets rich in antioxidants and fibre, which not only aided her recovery but also invigorated her entrepreneurial spirit. With every healthy meal, Maria felt stronger and more in control of her body, inspiring her to share her newfound knowledge through workshops for other women facing similar challenges.

Another remarkable journey is that of Angela, who turned her health struggles into a passion for holistic nutrition. After her surgery, she delved deeply into research on foods that help balance hormones and reduce inflammation. Angela created a personalised meal plan that incorporated nourishing ingredients like leafy greens, whole grains, and healthy fats. Her commitment to her diet transformed her recovery experience and reignited her ambition to launch a business dedicated to helping other women embrace nutritious lifestyles for better health. Through her journey, Angela exemplifies how adversity can lead to new opportunities and a purpose-driven life.

The story of Lisa is a testament to the power of community and support. After her myomectomy, she found solace in a group of women who shared their experiences and recovery strategies. Together, they explored nutrition, participated in cooking classes, and held each other accountable in their health journeys. Lisa discovered that healing is not just an individual endeavor but a collective experience. Through this supportive network, she learned the importance of nurturing relationships as part of her recovery, which helped her maintain a positive mindset and stay committed to her health goals.

These inspiring journeys illustrate that recovery from a myomectomy is not merely about physical healing but also about embracing a holistic approach to well-being. Women like Maria, Angela, and Lisa demonstrate that with the right mindset, education, and support, it is possible to thrive after surgery. By prioritizing nutrition and building a community around shared experiences, they have rewritten their narratives, proving that the path to a fibroid-free life is paved with empowerment, resilience, and hope.

Lessons Learned from Others

In the journey towards fibroid-free living, the experiences of others can serve as powerful sources of inspiration and guidance. Many women have faced the challenges of fibroid surgery and the fear of recurrence. By examining their stories, we can uncover valuable lessons that empower us to take control of our health and well-being. These narratives highlight the importance of proactive measures, such as nutrition and lifestyle changes, which can significantly impact recovery and long-term health.

One common thread among those who have successfully navigated the post-myomectomy landscape is the emphasis on dietary choices. Women report transformative results after adopting nutrient-dense diets rich in whole foods, healthy fats, and lean proteins. By prioritising foods that reduce inflammation and support hormonal balance, they have not only improved their overall health but have also actively worked against the regrowth of fibroids. These lessons remind us that what we consume plays a crucial role in our recovery and can be a powerful tool for prevention.

Moreover, the power of community cannot be underestimated. Many women have found solace and strength in connecting with others who share similar experiences. Support groups and online forums provide a platform for exchanging tips, recipes, and encouragement. Hearing the success stories of others who have embraced nutrition and made lifestyle adjustments can motivate us to stick to our goals. This collective wisdom reinforces the idea that we are not alone in our journey; we can learn from each other and uplift one another.

Another lesson learned from these remarkable women is the importance of listening to our bodies. Many shared their struggles with adhering to strict diets or exercise regimens but eventually discovered the significance of tuning into their own needs. By cultivating self-awareness and understanding how their bodies respond to different foods and activities, they were able to create personalized plans that suited their lifestyles. This lesson teaches us that flexibility and self-compassion are vital components of any recovery journey.

Lastly, resilience emerges as a prominent theme in the stories of those who have thrived after myomectomy. The road to recovery is often filled with setbacks, but many women have demonstrated that persistence and a positive mindset can lead to remarkable outcomes. By learning from the challenges faced by others and embracing a proactive approach to nutrition and self-care, we can foster our own resilience. Every step taken towards better health is a step towards empowerment, and the lessons learned from others illuminate the path to a fibroid-free future.

The Power of Community Support

The journey of recovery after a myomectomy can be daunting, but the power of community support can transform this experience into one of empowerment and hope. For professional and entrepreneurial women navigating the complexities of post-surgery life, connecting with others who share similar challenges can provide invaluable encouragement. This sense of community supports a safe space where women can share their experiences, exchange practical advice, and uplift one another through the healing process.

Engaging with a supportive network not only alleviates feelings of isolation but also reinforces the importance of nutrition and wellness in preventing fibroid regrowth. In these communities, women often discover that they are not alone in their struggles and that others have successfully navigated the same path. This shared knowledge can be a powerful tool in developing personalised nutrition and diet plans that cater specifically to post-myomectomy recovery. The exchange of recipes, meal prep strategies, and tips on maintaining a balanced diet becomes a collective effort that strengthens individual resolve.

Moreover, community support often extends beyond the realm of food and nutrition. It can encompass emotional and mental well-being, both of which are crucial during recovery. Women can find strength in each other's stories, drawing inspiration from those who have overcome similar obstacles. The encouragement that comes from a community can motivate individuals to prioritise self-care and wellness, reinforcing the idea that healing is not just a physical journey but also an emotional one.

As members of these communities share their triumphs and setbacks, they create a rich collage of experiences that can lead to deeper understanding and compassion. This environment nurtures resilience, empowering women to take control of their health and well-being. It is in these circles that they learn about holistic approaches to nutrition and how lifestyle choices play a pivotal role in preventing the recurrence of fibroids. The shared commitment to maintaining a fibroid-free life becomes a collective mission infused with hope and determination.

Undoubtedly, the power of community support lies in its ability to inspire and motivate women to advocate for their health. By building connections with others who are on similar journeys, women and cultivates a sense of empowerment that propels them toward sustainable lifestyle changes. Together, they can champion the importance of nutrition, share resources, and celebrate successes, reinforcing the belief that they have the strength to thrive beyond surgery and embrace a fibroid-free future.

CHAPTER 10

MOVING FORWARD WITH CONFIDENCE

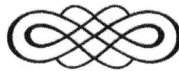

Celebrating Your Progress

Celebrating your progress is an essential part of the journey toward healing and empowerment after a myomectomy. As women who are dedicated to navigating the complexities of recovery while managing the demands of professional and entrepreneurial life, recognising the strides you have made can provide motivation and reinforce your commitment to a fibroid-free future. Each small victory, whether it is successfully incorporating a new nutritious recipe into your diet or feeling more energetic throughout your day, deserves acknowledgment. These celebrations not only boost your morale but also serve as reminders of your strength and resilience.

Tracking your progress can take many forms, from maintaining a journal to documenting your nutritional choices and their effects on your well-being. Reflecting on how far you have come helps you appreciate the positive changes you are making in your life. Consider setting specific milestones related to your nutrition and lifestyle changes, such as sticking to a meal plan for a month or achieving a personal goal of incorporating more plant-based meals into your diet. Each milestone reached is an opportunity to celebrate your commitment to your health and can inspire you to continue prioritising your well-being.

Incorporating community into your celebration amplifies the joy of your progress. Sharing your achievements with friends, family, or a support group creates a sense of accountability and connection. It is empowering to surround yourself with like-minded women who understand the challenges of post-myomectomy recovery. Consider organising a small gathering or virtual meet-up where you can share recipes, discuss experiences, and celebrate one another's successes. This camaraderie not only reinforces your commitment but also fosters a supportive environment where everyone can thrive.

Do not underestimate the power of self-care in your journey. Celebrating your progress can also mean treating yourself to something special, whether it is a spa day, a new book on nutrition, or a cooking class that focuses on healthy meals. These rewards can rejuvenate your spirit and remind you that your journey toward health is as much about enjoyment as it is about discipline. By prioritising self-care, you reinforce the idea that investing in your health is a worthy endeavor, and you are deserving of these moments of joy and relaxation.

As you continue on this path, keep in mind that the journey is not solely about the destination but the growth and learning you experience along the way. Each step you take toward a healthier lifestyle contributes to a future free from the burden of fibroids and a dependance on strong medication. Embrace and celebrate your progress, big or small, and let it empower you to forge ahead with renewed vigor. Your dedication to nurturing your body through nutrition and mindful living is a testament to your strength, and each celebration is a powerful reminder of the positive impact you are making in your life.

Setting Future Health Goals

Setting future health goals is a crucial step for professional and entrepreneurial women who have undergone a myomectomy. Understanding the journey ahead can empower you to take control of your health and well-being. By emphasising the importance of setting clear, achievable goals, you can create a roadmap that not only prevents the regrowth of fibroids but also enhances your overall quality of life. This proactive approach will enable you to thrive in your personal and professional endeavors while prioritising your health.

Begin by defining what health means to you post-surgery. Consider the specific outcomes you desire, whether it is maintaining a healthy weight, boosting energy levels, or achieving hormonal balance. Reflect on how these goals align with your lifestyle, family, and professional commitments. By establishing a personal vision of health, you can create a foundation that supports both your physical and emotional well-being. This tailored approach ensures that your goals resonate with your individual circumstances, making them more attainable and meaningful.

Next, develop a nutrition and diet plan that aligns with your health goals. Focus on incorporating whole, nutrient-dense foods that support recovery and prevent fibroid regrowth. Emphasise the importance of low sugary fruits, vegetables, organic lean proteins, and healthy fats in your daily meals. By prioritising a balanced diet, you not only nourish your body but also promote resilience against potential womb challenges. Consider meal prepping and planning as essential tools to help you stay on track, even amidst a busy schedule. This commitment to nutrition will empower you to make informed choices that benefit your long-term health.

In addition to nutrition, incorporate regular physical activity into your routine. Find exercises that you enjoy, whether it is yoga, pilates, or brisk walking. Engaging in physical activity not only helps manage stress but also supports hormonal balance and overall wellness. Set realistic fitness goals, such as dedicating a certain number of days each week to exercise. Celebrate your progress along the way, regardless of how small, as this will reinforce your commitment to a healthier lifestyle and keep you motivated.

Finally, remember that setting future health goals is an ongoing process. Regularly reassess your goals and adjust as needed. Life is dynamic, and as you evolve in your personal and professional journey, so will your health aspirations. Surround yourself with a supportive community, whether through friends, family, or health professionals, who encourage you in your quest for optimal health. By staying committed to your goals and embracing each step of the journey, you will not only embody a fibroid-free life but also inspire others to pursue their health and wellness ambitions.

Embracing a Fibroid-Free Lifestyle

Embracing a fibroid-free lifestyle is not just about recovery; it is a powerful commitment to your overall well-being. As professional and entrepreneurial women, your lives are filled with responsibilities, ambitions, and dreams. It is essential to remember that prioritising your health is a crucial part of your journey. Adopting a lifestyle that supports fibroid-free living empowers you to take control of your body and future. This means incorporating mindful eating, regular physical activity, and stress management techniques into your daily routine. By doing so, you are not only fostering your recovery but also enhancing your overall quality of life.

Nutrition plays a pivotal role in preventing the regrowth of fibroids. After a myomectomy, focusing on a balanced diet rich in whole foods significantly impacts your healing. Emphasise foods that are high in fibre, such as fruits low in sugars, vegetables, and whole grains, as they aid digestion and hormone regulation. Incorporating lean organic proteins, healthy fats, and a variety of vitamins and minerals will provide the necessary nutrients for recovery and optimal health. Remember, the choices you make today will set the foundation for a healthier tomorrow, reducing the risk of fibroid recurrence consistency is key.

In addition to nutrition, regular physical activity is vital in maintaining a fibroid-free lifestyle. Engaging in exercises that you enjoy helps to keep your body strong and resilient. Consider activities such as hot yoga, pilates, or brisk walking, which not only strengthen the body but also promote relaxation and stress relief. By integrating movement into your daily routine, you will enhance circulation, support hormonal balance, and improve your mood. This holistic approach to fitness will empower you to tackle challenges with renewed energy, both personally and professionally.

Stress management is another critical component of a fibroid-free lifestyle. As busy women, it is easy to let stress accumulate, but it is essential to find effective ways to manage it. Techniques such as mindfulness meditation, deep breathing exercises, or even journaling can help you process your thoughts and emotions. Prioritise self-care by carving out time for activities that bring you joy and peace. By nurturing your mental and emotional well-being, you create a supportive environment for your physical health, making it less likely for fibroids to return.

Finally, connecting with a supportive community can make all the difference in your journey. Surround yourself with women who understand your experiences and can provide encouragement and inspiration. Whether through support groups, online forums, or social media, sharing your journey and learning from others offer invaluable insights. Embracing a fibroid-free lifestyle is not just a personal commitment; it is a collective movement towards empowerment and healing. As you move forward, remember that you are not alone, and your choices today are paving the way for a healthier, fibroid-free future.

ABOUT THE AUTHOR

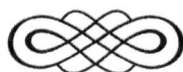

Nina Lemtir is a passionate advocate for women's womb health, a successful entrepreneur, and a living testament to the power of holistic healing. After nearly losing her womb to fibroids and enduring multiple miscarriages, Nina commenced on a life changing journey to reclaim her health. By blending lifestyle changes, nutrition, and a commitment to self-care, she not only overcame her own struggles but also welcomed three beautiful children into her life.

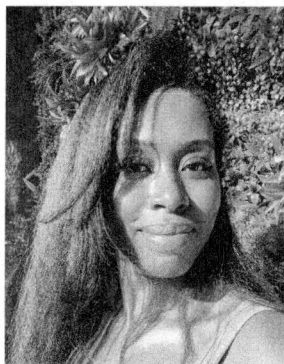

As a former salon owner, Nina understands the toll of balancing ambition with personal well-being. Her first-hand experience with ignoring debilitating symptoms while prioritising her career led her to write *Beyond the Surgery*, a heartfelt and empowering guide for women battling fibroids. In her book, she sheds light on alternative approaches to healing, offering hope and actionable solutions beyond the repeated cycles of surgery.

Today, Nina is the founder of a groundbreaking program dedicated to helping women shrink fibroids naturally, avoid unnecessary hysterectomies, and take control of their fertility. Her mission is to inspire women to advocate for themselves, explore holistic solutions, and lead fulfilling lives despite the challenges of womb disorders.

Through *Beyond the Surgery* and her workshops, Nina shares her story to let women know they are not alone—and that healing is possible.

Weekly Meal Planning

Instructions:
- Use this template to track your meals, snacks, and beverages.
- Note number and symptoms or how you feel after each meal to identify patterns.
- Stay hydrated plus electrolytes and aim for a balanced diet rich in whole foods vegetables, low sugar fruits, whole grains, and organic plant-based proteins.

Week:_____   Month:_____

MONDAY
Breakfast:	Water: ① ② ③ ④ ⑤	Notes
Lunch:	Vitamins: ① ② ③ ④ ⑤	
Dinner:	Veggies: ① ② ③ ④ ⑤	
Snack:	Symptoms: ① ② ③ ④ ⑤	

TUESDAY
Breakfast:	Water: ① ② ③ ④ ⑤	Notes
Lunch:	Vitamins: ① ② ③ ④ ⑤	
Dinner:	Veggies: ① ② ③ ④ ⑤	
Snack:	Symptoms: ① ② ③ ④ ⑤	

WEDNESDAY
Breakfast:	Water: ① ② ③ ④ ⑤	Notes
Lunch:	Vitamins: ① ② ③ ④ ⑤	
Dinner:	Veggies: ① ② ③ ④ ⑤	
Snack:	Symptoms: ① ② ③ ④ ⑤	

THURSDAY
Breakfast:	Water: ① ② ③ ④ ⑤	Notes
Lunch:	Vitamins: ① ② ③ ④ ⑤	
Dinner:	Veggies: ① ② ③ ④ ⑤	
Snack:	Symptoms: ① ② ③ ④ ⑤	

FRIDAY
Breakfast:	Water: ① ② ③ ④ ⑤	Notes
Lunch:	Vitamins: ① ② ③ ④ ⑤	
Dinner:	Veggies: ① ② ③ ④ ⑤	
Snack:	Symptoms: ① ② ③ ④ ⑤	

SATURDAY
Breakfast:	Water: ① ② ③ ④ ⑤	Notes
Lunch:	Vitamins: ① ② ③ ④ ⑤	
Dinner:	Veggies: ① ② ③ ④ ⑤	
Snack:	Symptoms: ① ② ③ ④ ⑤	

SUNDAY
Breakfast:	Water: ① ② ③ ④ ⑤	Notes
Lunch:	Vitamins: ① ② ③ ④ ⑤	
Dinner:	Veggies: ① ② ③ ④ ⑤	
Snack:	Symptoms: ① ② ③ ④ ⑤	

Notes

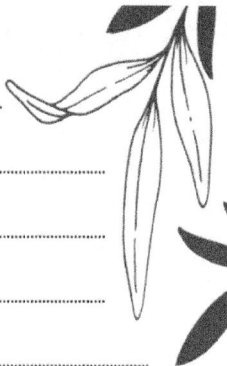

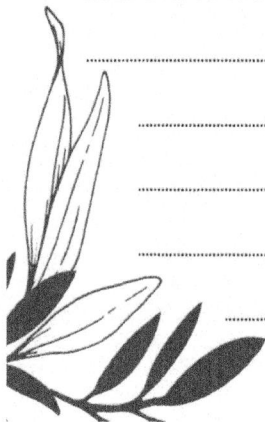

Notes

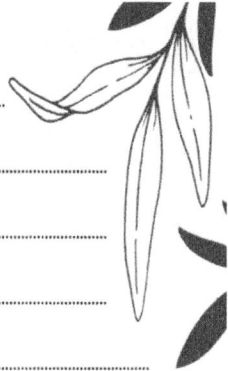
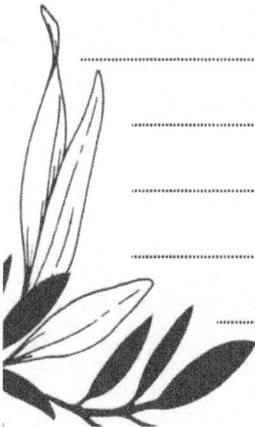

Notes

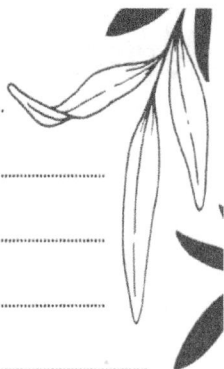
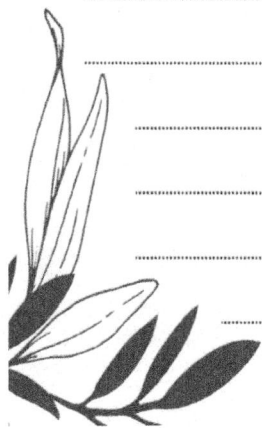

Printed in Great Britain
by Amazon

62406785R00070